get the
sugar
out

get the sugar out

501 SIMPLE WAYS TO CUT THE SUGAR OUT OF ANY DIET

Completely Updated and Revised 2nd Edition

Ann Louise Gittleman, Ph.D., C.N.S.

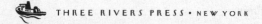
THREE RIVERS PRESS • NEW YORK

Three Rivers Press and the Tugboat design are registered trademarks
of Random House, Inc.

Originally published in different form by Three Rivers Press,
an imprint of the Crown Publishing Group, a division of
Random House, Inc., New York, in 1996.

Permissions to reprint already published recipes appear on pages 267–74.

Library of Congress Cataloging-in-Publication Data

Gittleman, Ann Louise.
    Get the sugar out : 501 simple ways to cut the sugar out of any
diet / Ann Louise Gittleman.—2nd ed.
        p. cm.
    Includes bibliographical references and index.
    1. Sugar-free diet.   I. Title.
    RM237.85.G55 2008
    613.2'8—dc22   2007023873

ISBN 978-0-307-39485-9

Printed in the United States of America

Design by Kay Schuckhart / Blond on Pond

10 9 8 7 6 5

Second Edition

This book is dedicated to Isaac Aaron Gittleman,
a beloved addition to the Gittleman family

acknowledgments

I would like to acknowledge the creative team at Crown Publishers for their strong support of this newly revised book. My deepest thanks go to my editor, Lindsey Moore; copy editor Sue Warga; production editor Cindy Berman; publicist Jennifer Reyes; publishing manager Carrie Thornton, and, of course, my literary agent, Coleen O'Shea, for making this all happen in the first place! Once upon a time, Coleen was my editor for my very first book. So, literally and figuratively, she deserves my gratitude and profound thanks for spearheading my writing career. Thank you, Coleen!

I am also grateful for the research and creative work that Kathryn Winifred Mays Wright, M.A., contributed to this project. Katey was always there for last-minute fact-checks, and I so appreciate her sterling work ethic and grace under pressure. I hope we will work together again, Katey.

My personal thanks to Stuart Gittleman, my significant brother, who is also the operations and business manager of First Lady of Nutrition, Inc. Stuart inherited our father's wonderful sense of humor, patience, and objectivity. He has handled all of our business dealings with a great deal of sensitivity and integrity. I am very proud of him!

I also must acknowledge my personal assistant Tami Oliver, the most focused organizer and planner this side of the Mississippi. Tami has kept my office, my files, and my closet "together" through a very hectic year of writing and personal challenges—without batting an eyelash. You are a true "woman of valor," Ms. Tami.

Speaking of "women of valor," I simply must mention my circle of women associates, friends, and professionals (many of whom are all three) who have been especially supportive of me during the updating of this book. It has been very comforting knowing that I have such a resource of wonderful women when I need them. Thanks to all these lovely ladies for being there: Liz Krichman, Susan Meredith, Linda Hooper, Dr. Shirley Scott, my cousin Donna Lee, Dr. Nan Fuchs, Siri Khalsa, Roon Frost, Jo Len Schoor, Vicki Accardi, Susan Carlson, Jeannette Boudreau, Kathryn McKinley, Anne Hiaring, Sally Manthos, Lena Coleman, Jolie Root, Frankie Boyer, Judy Williams, Dr. Nancy, Joan Lanning, Chee Chee Phillips, Laura Evenson, Christina Long, Llolyn Pobram, Kathie Moe, Judi Wilson, Karen Jarmon, and my mother, Edith Gittleman.

Finally, there are several very special men whom I would like to recognize: Dr. Brad Reed and Dr. Paul Schutz (my chiropractors), Dr. Kevin Johnson, Rex Lettau (my trainer), Howard M. Lee (my acupuncturist), and most of all James William Templeton, the love of my life.

contents

get the
sugar
out

sugar savvy 101: the facts about sugar and its kissing cousins

*a*s you have probably heard, all of us should be eating less sugar. Here's why: Sugar has been linked to more than sixty different ailments, including obesity. While refined sugar consumption has declined in recent years, a new breed of sugar substitutes has emerged in the form of artificial sweeteners such as Splenda, aspartame, and sugar alcohols, as well as high-fructose corn syrup (HFCS). Alarmingly, sugar's "kissing cousins" may be even more harmful to your health than sugar itself.

So today it is more important than ever that you understand and practice *sugar savvy*.

HFCS is perhaps the most insidious of all sugar substitutes, as it alone accounts for more than 40 percent of caloric sweeteners added to foods and drinks in the United States—with consumption growth matching the escalating rise in obesity. Did you know that between 1970 and 2000 per capita consumption of HFCS in the United States went from an estimated 0.6 pounds per person per year to a whopping 73.5 pounds, according to figures from the U.S. Department of Agricultural Economic Research Service?

You might see a label that doesn't list the white stuff and think that you are home free. Not true. Manufacturers are now using the cheaper HFCS and artificial sweeteners to take the place of sugar, and both artificial sweeteners and HFCS have been implicated in the fattening of America. (For more information on the dangers of artificial sweeteners, see the **"Consumer Alert: What You Need to Know About the Top Two Artificial Sugar Substitutes"** on page 55.)

The perception of "sugar-free" is not unlike that of "fat-free" in the 1980s and early 1990s. Consider this: Ever since we started slashing the fat and consuming those monster-sized low-fat muffins and boxes of fat-free cookies—you remember the Snack-Well's craze—we have actually gotten fatter, going from a 25 percent obesity rate in the 1970s to more than double that two decades later. Why? Because Americans were consuming those fat-free goodies with abandon, disregarding the fact that they usually have *more* sugar, and sometimes only slightly fewer calories, than the original products.

Let's take a close look at Nabisco Fig Newtons cookies as an example. Two of the original Fig Newtons supply you with 13 grams of sugars and 110 calories. If you eat two Nabisco Fat-Free Fig Newtons, thinking you're doing your body a favor, you'll get no fat, but you'll get more sugar—15 grams instead of 13 grams— and only 10 fewer calories.

Add to this the fact that the fat in the original cookie helps satiate your appetite, so you are apt to eat only a few. With the fat-free kind, people sometimes eat whole boxes without ever feeling satisfied.

Nonetheless, sales of fat-free products skyrocketed. In line with this modern misconception (or should I say health deception?), reduced-sugar products now line the shelves and ultimately play this same trick on your hunger receptors and your waistline. Consider that roughly a decade ago 36 reduced-sugar products had edged their way into your local supermarket. In 2003 that number jumped to 607. In 2004 about 2,200 sugarless or sugar-reduced products were available for sale in the United States. Reduced-sugar and sugar-free products, from breakfast cereals to jelly beans, have taken up permanent residence on our supermarket shelves. And they are multiplying rapidly. So before you automatically reach for that reduced-sugar product, remind yourself that it is up to *you* to be your own food detective.

As a food detective, you simply need to recognize that if you are automatically reaching for a product advertising itself as "reduced-sugar" to be able to eat sweets without the intake of calories, you may be in for a rude awakening. When a product is supplemented with one of sugar's kissing cousins you may not be significantly reducing calories at all. For example in 2003, Jelly Belly jelly beans added Splenda to decrease the sugar content and slapped on a "sugar-free" label. Yet the difference between the original Jelly Belly and the sugar-free Jelly Belly is *only one calorie.*

Finally, as a food detective, you need to ask yourself whether or not sugar substitutes are really safe. In fact, the sugar substitute in our example—Splenda—has been linked to a variety of symptoms such as headaches, bloating, and stomach cramps. Consider that the official Jelly Belly Web site warns that children under three years of age should not consume the sugar-free kinds because their immature digestive system combined with smaller body mass could trigger digestive discomfort, and suggests that parents should carefully monitor children's total consumption.

As a matter of fact, a number of studies suggest that consumption of artificial sweeteners can actually increase caloric intake. For example, after eight years of collecting data, Sharon P. Fowler, MPH, and her colleagues reported the results of a study conducted at the University of Texas Health Sciences Center noting a 41 percent increase in risk of being overweight for every can or bottle of diet soft drink a person consumes each day.* The moral of this study: Remember to not only watch what you eat—watch what you *drink.*

I believe the low-carb craze of the 1990s is to blame for the enormous amount of artificial sweeteners, especially sugar alcohols, in so many foods. The consumption of artificial sweeteners, in the form of sugar alcohols such as mannitol, sorbitol, and xylitol (see tip 56) may increase caloric intake. Made popular during the low-carb craze (think of all those low-carb protein bars and shakes), sugar alcohols originate from fruits and berries and so they seem "natural" enough. But more insidious, sugar-alcohol-laced low-carb goodies are touted by manufacturers as being virtually "sugar-free" (sugar alcohols are not technically really sugar) because of the perception that the calories or sugars in these foods don't count.

Why? The carbs from sugar alcohols metabolize into glucose much more slowly than real sugar and so don't impact blood

*Sharon P. Fowler, Abstract 1058-P, 65th Annual Scientific Sessions, American Diabetes Association, San Diego, June 10–14, 2005.

sugar levels the way sugar does. In light of this concept, manufacturers subtract the sugar alcohols from a product's total amount of carbs, and what is left is known as "net carbs."

With people under the impression that low-carb foods are also low-calorie because the sugar alcohols in the products don't really count as carbs, low-carb food sales soared. But the sad reality is that sugar alcohols do raise glucose levels in the blood. Just ask the American Diabetes Association. You need to consider *all* the carbs and *all* the calories in any sugar-alcohol-containing product and ignore the deceptive "net carb" label.

Even more worrisome is the reality that there are not enough clinical trials on sugar alcohols to warrant their safe use.

It certainly appears that sugar and friends may be one of the root causes of our obesity epidemic and associated health problems, much more so than fat, that maligned and misunderstood nutrient, which in the recent past was considered the dietary boogeyman. Just for the record, let me say that I strongly believe that the fear of eating fat can make you fat, as I discuss in practically all of my twenty-five books, including my *New York Times* bestseller, *The Fat Flush Plan.* The bottom line here is that the right kind of fat is an essential nutrient that our bodies need; sugar and company, on the other hand, are *something we don't need at all.*

Statistics in France seem to prove this. Even though the French diet is higher in fat than the American diet, the French are much less afflicted by obesity and heart disease than Americans are. What's the French secret to maintaining weight and better health? It appears to be that in France, per capita sugar consumption is roughly *five and a half times less* than that in America. Humans don't require sugar, yet average Americans consume their body weight in sugar each year.

If all Americans knew the dangers of sugar, it would be withdrawn from our list of safe food additives. Refined sugar acts more like a drug that our bodies must detoxify rather than a nutrient-supplying food. Refined sugar is, in fact, nutrientless. Important nutrients such as chromium, manganese, cobalt, copper, zinc, and magnesium are stripped away in sugar refining, and our bodies actually have to use their own mineral reserves just to digest it. With lots of calories but no nutrients, sugar and its substitutes are the number one cause of America's lack of nutrition—a combination known as *overconsumptive malnutrition.* What this term basically means is that Americans are consuming too many calories that add up in weight but don't give us the nutrients we need to keep our bodies functioning properly. Imagine malnutrition in America in this day and age!

Our distant ancestors ate no concentrated sugars. Even in the infancy of this country, people ate sugar only as a rare treat. But now sugar and other sweeteners have become part of our everyday diet. Little by little, as our country has developed and become more "civilized," Americans have become more and more "sugarized." The chart on page 7 shows the alarming rise in sugar consumption in America since the early 1800s.

And things have gotten worse—the average person today eats about 180 pounds of sugar per year, or around ½ pound of sugar per day. Compare this to the consumption of less than 10 pounds of sugar per year in the late 1700s and you can see that *sugar consumption has risen more than 1,800 percent in the last two hundred years!*

As alluded to earlier, there is another cause for concern, and that is the overuse of high-fructose corn syrup (HFCS). The truth

Approximate Sugar Consumption per Person Each Year	
YEAR	AMOUNT IN POUNDS
Early 1800s	12
1850	22
1875	41
1895	63
1915	95
1935	115
1955	119
1976	125
1990	130–40
1996	153
1999	158
2006	180

is that HFCS is a concentrated sweetener your brain doesn't even recognize as a sugar. By replacing sugar with HFCS, you can override your body's natural ability to feel full, so you eat more. Without this type of signal you don't know when to stop eating. Now that is downright scary.

HFCS is found in just about every food in our supermarket, including sodas, juices, candies, syrups, pasta sauces, cookies, cakes, energy bars, baked goods, canned foods, salad dressing, breakfast cereals, yogurt, ketchup, frozen foods, baby formula, and more.

The consumption of HFCS increased an incredible 1,000 percent from 1970 to 1990 alone. In fact, today the average consumption of all corn sweeteners, including HFCS, is 83 pounds per year. (To learn even more about HFCS in relation to your growing waistline, see "Obesity" on page 23.)

Such a drastic change in the human diet in less than two cen-

Estimated per Capita Sweetener Consumption, Total and by Type of Sweetener, 1966–2004

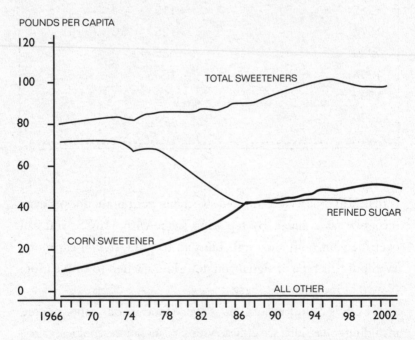

Stephen Haley, Jane Reed, Biing-Hwan Lin, and Annetta Cook, *Sweetener Consumption in the United States: Distribution by Demographic and Product Characteristic,* Electronic Outlook Report from the Economic Research Service; United States Department of Agriculture SSS-243-01, www.ers.usda.gov, August 2005.

turies is a cause for great concern. Evolutionary changes occur over hundreds of thousands of years; the human body of today is still very similar to the Stone Age model of forty thousand years ago. To change the kinds of calories consumed by humans so dramatically in so short a time is an invitation to trouble. Our bodies simply haven't had time to respond and adapt to this nutrient-poor source of calories—and it appears that our bodies are rebelling with a multitude of physical ailments, telling us loudly and clearly that they don't like what they're being fed.

We all know sugar causes dental cavities, but recent evidence has also shown that sugar is associated with weakened immunity, heart disease, high blood pressure, cancer, obesity, metabolic syndrome, aging, and more. (For a complete list of the ailments associated with sugar consumption, see "The Problems with Sugar," page 16.) We also know without a doubt that excess calories from sugar and HFCS can readily turn into body fat. Remember that the next time you catch yourself thinking that "fat-free" translates into "eat all you want."

Many of you are already well aware that sugar is harmful to your health and are eager to move on to the tips, so I won't mince words. Fat, like protein, is an essential nutrient for human health. *Simple sugars are not!* We could live very nicely (much better, in fact) if we never ate another ounce of sugar.

If you would like to understand the intricate details of *why* that statement is true, keep on reading. If you do decide to skip the next section and move directly on to the tips right now, I recommend that you come back to the important information that follows when you have more time. Knowing exactly why we should avoid sugar helps instill a much deeper resolve to reduce our sugar intake.

understanding sugar

The term *sugar* can be misleading.

Most of us hear the word and think of table sugar, the end product of the refining of sugarcane. But the term can be used in so many different contexts and have so many different meanings that confusion abounds. (Food manufacturers couldn't be happier about this confusion because they often use it to their advantage.)

To understand what sugar really is, you first have to understand some basics about carbohydrates. Carbohydrates are one of three energy-producing nutrients our bodies need; the other two are protein and fat. As a fuel, carbohydrates are the cleanest-burning of the three and the best provider of glucose, a fuel our muscles need for get-up-and-go and a fuel our brains need for clear thinking and steady behavior.

There are two significantly different types of carbohydrates, simple and complex. Simple carbohydrates, which consist of one or two sugar units in every molecule, are also known as *simple sugars*. They supply virtually instant energy for the body, but they don't provide energy that lasts. As you might have guessed, table sugar (also known as dextrose or sucrose) is one type of simple sugar. But so are natural sweeteners such as honey and molasses; fructose, which is found naturally in fruits and can also be a sweetener; and lactose, which is a naturally occurring sugar found in dairy products. (For a complete list of different types of simple sugars, see tip 79.) Complex carbohydrates, on the other hand, are made up of long chains of simple sugars. As their name implies, they are much more complex in structure than simple sugars and require longer digestion to be absorbed. This is beneficial in the long run because the sugars they contain are released more slowly and gradually in the bloodstream, supplying steadier, longer-lasting energy for the body. Complex carbohydrates are found in starches (whole grains and starchy vegetables such as potatoes), legumes (such as beans and peas), and vegetables (such as lettuce, broccoli, and zucchini). These are really good examples of *hidden sugars* in your diet.

Lately we have heard much about the value of eliminating bad carbohydrates in our diet, but we still make little distinction between the two kinds. Avoiding vegetables and starches and munching on sugar-laden muffins, cookies, and candy, even if they are low-fat, is not the way we should meet our carbohydrate needs, yet it is the way more and more of us are choosing to eat. At the beginning of the last century, two-thirds of the carbohydrates eaten by Americans came from complex sources such as potatoes, vegetables, and grains. *Today, amazingly, half of all carbohydrates consumed come from simple sugars.* These statistics confirm what we already know: We are becoming sugarholics.

What the statistics don't show, however, is equally important to understand. Most of the "complex" carbohydrates Americans consume aren't really that complex after all. Although classified as complex carbohydrates (because they're made from grains, not sugars), white pasta, bread, and bagels really react more like simple sugars in the body because the flour in them is highly refined. In refining, nutrient- and fiber-rich whole grains are converted into processed foods that have a long shelf life but many calories and few nutrients (sometimes as much as 86 percent less of some nutrients than are in the original grain). Nutritionally, there is little difference between processed carbohydrates and simple sugars. In fact, far from being healthy foods, these processed carbohydrates contribute to blood sugar problems, weight gain, and malnutrition and give us little in return. You should think of processed carbohydrates as hidden sugars in the diet. (They're "hidden" because they are disguised as complex carbohydrates.)

When either sugars or processed carbohydrates are eaten, they are broken down almost immediately, and a flood of sugar is released directly into the bloodstream. In response to so much sugar, the pancreas secretes insulin, a hormone that is designed to restore blood sugar equilibrium by taking excess sugar out of the bloodstream and either transforming it into glycogen for energy for our muscles or moving it into fat storage. But the human body was never designed to deal with so many concentrated sweeteners, so the pancreas ends up doing its job too well. In response to excess sugar in the bloodstream, the pancreas produces so much insulin that blood sugar drops too low. The result is a quick burst of energy followed by an equally fast drop in energy. At the same time, insulin causes sugar removed from the bloodstream to be stored as body fat instead. Once you understand these basic nutrition principles, you can see how fat-free (but sugar- and processed-carbohydrate-rich) goodies are *not* the way to lose weight or to provide any kind of long-term energy.

To understand sugars and carbohydrates and the insulin response to them, it's also extremely helpful to know about the glycemic index of foods. The glycemic index is a listing based upon real-life blood sugar levels after the ingestion of various foods. Low-glycemic-index foods rank between 0 and 40 on the scale (the reference point is glucose, at 100) and raise the blood sugar slowly and gradually. They are the least likely to cause blood sugar fluctuations, followed, of course, by moderate-glycemic-index foods. High-glycemic-index foods, however, cause an alarmingly fast rise in blood sugar, followed by an equally severe blood sugar crash. In other words, they are high inducers of insulin secretion.

To help you understand the glycemic index, keep in mind three things:

1. Foods that rank lower on the index help maintain weight, balance blood sugar, and give better, longer-term energy than higher-index foods, which give quick bursts of energy. Put simply, less is more.

2. Eating some protein or fat with moderate- or high-glycemic-index foods helps to slow down the body's insulin response and keep blood sugar more steady.

3. Even when they rank equally with whole-grain products on the glycemic index, processed carbohydrates such as white pasta are still less desirable than whole-grain products because they lack vitamins, minerals, and fiber.

Once you understand the structure and different kinds of sugar and the body's glycemic response, you can understand why sugar harms your health.

The following list is a sampling of common foods in each category you can use as a general guide.*

To find out the glycemic index value of a certain food or to learn more on this topic, check out the searchable database on the Web site www.glycemicindex.com.

---

*The Glycemic Index has been expanded upon and adapted from the *Nutritional Manual of BioFoods, Inc.*, of Santa Barbara, California. This chart was first developed by David Jenkins, M.D., Ph.D., professor of medicine and nutritional sciences at the University of Toronto.

The Glycemic Index of Foods

RAPID INDUCERS OF INSULIN

Glycemic index greater than 100
  Puffed rice
  Corn flakes
  Maltose
  Puffed wheat
  French baguette
  Instant white rice
  40 percent bran flakes
  Rice Krispies
  Weetabix
  Tofu ice-cream
    substitute
  Millet

Glycemic index of 100
  Glucose
  White bread
  Whole-wheat bread

Glycemic index between 90 and 99
  Grape-Nuts
  Carrots
  Parsnips
  Barley (whole-grain)

  Muesli
  Shredded wheat
  Apricots
  Corn chips

Glycemic index between 80 and 89
  Rolled oats
  Oat bran
  Honey
  White rice
  Brown rice
  White potato
  Corn
  Rye (whole-grain)
  Shortbread
  Ripe banana
  Ripe mango
  Ripe papaya

Glycemic index between 70 and 79
  All-Bran
  Kidney beans
  Wheat (coarse)
  Buckwheat
  Oatmeal cookies

The Glycemic Index of Foods

MODERATE INDUCERS OF INSULIN

Glycemic index between 60 and 69

Raisins

Mars candy bar

Spaghetti (white)

Spaghetti (whole-wheat)

Pinto beans

Macaroni

Pumpernickel bread

Bulgur

Couscous

Wheat kernels

Beets

Apple juice

Applesauce

Glycemic index between 50 and 59

Potato chips

Barley (pearl)

Green banana

Lactose

Peas (frozen)

Sucrose

Yam

Custard

Dried white beans

Glycemic index between 40 and 49

Sweet potato

Navy beans

Peas (dried)

Bran

Lima beans

Oatmeal (steel-cut)

Sponge cake

Butter beans

Grapes

Oranges

Orange juice

The Glycemic Index of Foods
REDUCED INSULIN SECRETION

Glycemic index between 30 and 39
- Apples
- Pears
- Tomato soup
- Ice cream
- Black-eyed peas
- Chickpeas
- Milk (skim)
- Milk (whole)
- Yogurt
- Fish sticks (breaded)

Glycemic index between 20 and 29
- Lentils
- Fructose

- Plums
- Peaches
- Grapefruit
- Cherries

Glycemic index between 10 and 19
- Soybeans
- Peanuts

the problems with sugar

Sugar has been blamed for nearly every known disease and even for the fall of several empires. While those accusations may sound like exaggerations, they probably are closer to the truth than you realize.

Saying sugar is bad for you is the ultimate understatement. The far-reaching problems sugar can cause are well documented in medical journals throughout the world, and new connections between sugar and disease are made each year.

Even as far back as the late 1960s and early 1970s—before I received my master's degree in nutrition—nutritional pioneers such as Adelle Davis, Carlton Fredericks, Dr. Herman Goodman, Dr. T. L. Cleave, and Dr. John Yudkin were already warning the public about the dangers of eating too much refined sugar. Twenty years earlier, Dr. E. M. Abrahamson, and A. W. Pezet wrote about the insulin connection to disease, the result of too much sugar in the diet. It is now more widely known than ever that sugar is bad. But how bad exactly?

CARDIOVASCULAR DISEASE

The sugar connection to heart disease was noticed in the 1970s. In the classic study *The Saccharine Disease* (Keats Publishing, 1975), T. L. Cleave showed convincing evidence that increases in cardiovascular disease, diabetes, and other common diseases could be traced to increases in sugar and refined carbohydrate intake. These diseases were virtually nonexistent in primitive cultures, he noted, until about twenty years after the societies began eating refined carbohydrates.

British researcher John Yudkin, M.D., came to a similar conclusion. In his classic book *Sweet and Dangerous* (Wyden Books, 1972), Dr. Yudkin cited numerous examples in a variety of societies that showed that sugar was a more likely cause of heart disease than fat. For example, the Masai and Samburu tribes of East Africa, he explained, have almost no heart disease, yet they eat a high-fat diet of mostly meat and milk—but no sugar. Recent research is proving the validity of the theories posed by Drs. Cleave and Yudkin, showing a direct relationship between sugar and heart disease because of insulin. Remember that when sugar is eaten, insulin is produced. Insulin not only helps to store excess sugar as fat (as explained before) but also helps regulate blood triglyceride levels, which are a major predictor of the development of heart disease. The more sugar you eat, the more insulin your pancreas will produce and the higher your triglyceride levels are likely to be.

High insulin levels in the blood are also linked to low levels of HDL cholesterol (the "good" cholesterol), high blood pressure, and obesity—three other important heart disease risk factors. Caused by the common problem of insulin resistance, this conglomeration of symptoms was originally named syndrome X in 1988 by Gerald Reaven, M.D., a world-renowned endocrinologist and professor emeritus at Stanford University School of Medicine. Today, this condition is more popularly known as prediabetes or metabolic syndrome (see more about this on page 19), and it probably affects 75 percent of Americans to some degree.

A number of books, such as *Syndrome X* by Jack Challem, Melissa Diane Smith, and Burton Berkson, have discussed how this condition may be the next public health crisis, silently afflicting people with the conditions previously mentioned as well as premature aging and degenerative diseases.

Could it be just a coincidence that at the same time the country was quietly being slipped HFCS in the general food supply, average cholesterol levels were going through the roof, not to mention the trend of increasing triglyceride levels and abnormal liver tests? How could this be? you ask. The answer is simple: Your body is not designed to metabolize HFCS. Put simply, the HFCS skips right past the need for insulin production, so your body doesn't send out a signal that it has eaten appetite-satisfying food. HFCS goes right into your cells, where it becomes an uncontrolled source of trouble all the way down to your liver. Your body just doesn't recognize HFCS, so it doesn't know how to control it, and in the end it becomes stored as fat (for more about this, see "Obesity" on page 23).

If you suspect metabolic syndrome, have your doctor perform some simple tests. Here are some things to look for:

- Low HDL levels (lower than 50 for men, lower than 60 for women)
- High triglycerides (greater than 100)
- High triglycerides/HDL ratio (greater than 4 to 1)
- Abnormal liver tests (AST, ALT, GGT)
- High serum ferritin (higher than 200)
- High serum uric acid (greater than 7)
- Low serum magnesium (lower than 2)
- Fasting blood sugar greater than 90
- Fasting insulin greater than 8

CANCER

As already noted, Americans consume on average of 180 pounds of sugar per person per year. According to Dr. Christine Horner in her book *Waking the Warrior Goddess,* "Cancer cells love sugar. It is their preferred fuel. The more sugar you eat, the faster cancer cells grow. Your pancreas responds to sugar by releasing insulin, the hormone that escorts sugar into your cells. When you eat refined simple sugars, such as table sugar, candy, cookies, or other sugar-laden foods, your blood sugar levels rise very quickly. Your pancreas responds by releasing a lot of insulin. That's not good. High insulin levels are one of the biggest risk factors and promoters of breast cancer. Women with high insulin levels have a 283 percent greater risk of breast cancer."

Horner goes on to explain that insulin attaches to breast cell receptors (healthy and/or cancerous), speeding up cell division in the same way estrogen does if it attaches to a receptor. And that's not all. Healthy levels of insulin naturally regulate the amount of estrogen that is available to attach to receptors, thereby naturally controlling excess estrogen-driven cell division. Understand that the cell division trouble created by excess insulin is twofold: more cancer and more healthy cells at risk for developing cancer.

As you might have guessed, excess sugar fuels the cancer fire in areas beyond breast tissue. One Swedish study with 80,000 participants documented that people who consume two or more carbonated drinks and/or use diluted sugar-sweetened fruit drinks a day have almost double the risk of developing pancreatic cancer.* Now consider that in 2004 Swedes drank an average of 76 liters of these kinds of beverages per year, while Americans averaged 200 liters per year.

As with heart disease, the prevalence of cancer has dramatically increased as America's (and other countries') sugar consumption has risen. While it's not clear whether sugar actually causes healthy cells to mutate and become cancerous, we do know one thing for sure: Once cells become cancerous, they feed directly on sugar, the way a yeast organism does during fermentation, and sugar can accelerate tumor growth.

---

*Susanna C. Larsson, Leif Bergkvist, and Alicja Wolk, "Consumption of sugar and sugar-sweetened foods and the risk of pancreatic cancer in a prospective study," *American Journal of Clinical Nutrition 84* (2006), 1171–6.

ADULT-ONSET DIABETES

Adult-onset diabetes, also known as type II diabetes, is another degenerative disease that has increased in frequency as sugar consumption has increased. Sugar's connection to this disease seems clear: During World War II, when sugar consumption in the United States dropped, the number of cases of adult-onset diabetes also dropped sharply.

This form of diabetes accounts for 98 percent of all the diabetes cases in America today and is considered to be almost entirely diet-related. It develops when insulin receptors in the cells no longer respond to the insulin being produced by the pancreas, and the cells are less able to get energy from the food we eat. Excess calories are then converted to fat, and numerous serious health complications can develop. Most health professionals agree that too many sugars and refined carbohydrates are at least a major contributing factor in the disease.

HYPOGLYCEMIA

Though diabetes is caused by high blood sugar, hypoglycemia is low blood sugar, a condition that often precedes the development of adult-onset diabetes. In hypoglycemia, the pancreas reacts to excess processed carbohydrates in the diet by sending out so much insulin that blood sugar drops too low, resulting in fatigue, lack of concentration, anxiety, mood swings, and irritability. Several health professionals, such as research psychologist Alexander Schauss, Ph.D., believe that alcoholics and drug addicts start out as hypoglycemics first and that hypoglycemia can also lead to criminal activity. Since almost all Americans eat too much sugar, many nutritionists think that most Americans are on an almost certain collision course with hypoglycemia.

AGING

I have already discussed how excess sugar raises insulin levels, which in turn speeds up the process of cell division, with consequences for cancer and elevated cancer risk. High insulin levels also negatively impact aging and life span. If you consider that, in theory, each of your cells is programmed to divide a finite number of times, with each division bringing the cell closer to death, then it is easy to understand why speeding up cell division speeds up aging. Eating sugar and sugar's kissing cousins is like pushing a fast-forward button on cellular age.

Just as we begin to understand that free radicals can deteriorate cells, scientists have confirmed that one of the most profound instruments of aging is a newly recognized aging by-product called advanced glycation end products or AGEs. AGEs are the result of a complicated chemical reaction involving the cross-linking of sugar and protein when your tissues are exposed to excess glucose. This effect has been described as "browning" because of the analogy between the glycation process and the browning effect that happens to the skin of a cooked turkey or chicken as the heated sugar becomes cross-linked with the heated protein. The glycation process changes the very structure of proteins.

In fact, the glycation process affects every organ in your body because collagen is one of the first proteins to be impacted. Collagen is the connective tissue that holds your skeleton, your muscles, and your blood vessels together. The first organs to show the effects of AGEs are your skin (think wrinkles and age spots), your immune system, and your eyes. While you may not be climbing into an oven anytime soon, the process the body goes through during normal metabolism also creates a kind of heating up of sugar and protein. So, throughout the course of your life, you are "cooking" from the inside out.

High levels of glucose have been shown to increase the production of both AGEs and free radicals, the highly unstable molecules that can damage cell membranes and start a chain reaction that can lead to chronic disease. Simply put, sugar can make you old before your time because the more sugar you consume, the more sugar your body must metabolize and the greater the amount of destructive by-products produced.

OBESITY

When high-fructose corn syrup became commonplace in the late 1970s, obesity levels began to soar. While the government has been offering subsidies to corn growers and there has been a savings of millions of dollars from the use of this cheaper sweetener, there has been a 100 percent increase in the rate of overweight and obesity in children and adolescents.

HFCS is a manmade, cheap, versatile, supersweet version of sucrose (aka table sugar). The problem is that it has introduced large quantities of a new *refined* version of fructose into the public food supply. While sucrose is 50 percent fructose and 50 percent glucose, HFCS is formed by adding specific enzymes to corn syrup in order to turn the high-glucose corn syrup into a 90 percent fructose product (HFCS 90). Then glucose is blended back in to get the desired glucose-fructose blend—usually 55 percent fructose and 45 percent glucose. Plus many filtration, ion exchange, and evaporation steps plus carbon adsorption (for removing impurities) are part of the process. Your body is not designed for high levels of *refined* fructose.

HFCS appears to affect our bodies differently than table sugar (sucrose). Every cell in your body can metabolize glucose, while the liver must metabolize fructose, so important appetite controls are bypassed. Unlike glucose, the fructose in HFCS is quickly absorbed into your cells without the help of insulin and without the subsequent increase in leptin, a hormone that regulates appetite by signaling to your brain that you are full. In addition, the insulin produced during glucose metabolism suppresses a hormone called ghrelin produced by the stomach to regulate food uptake; this action is missing with fructose metabolism, so you stay hungry and keep eating.

Plus fructose is metabolized differently by the liver than glucose; in fact, it is metabolized by a biochemical pathway in the liver that more easily leads to accumulation of body fat. So over time the cumulative effect of even a small increase in fructose combined with increased consumption adds up and adds pounds.

To add insult to injury, a study out of Perdue University offers support for the theory that artificial sweeteners increase caloric intake.* An unfortunate effect that these supersweet sugar substitutes are having on our bodies is a loss in our natural ability to "count" calories. Our bodies spent thousands of years developing the natural ability to estimate caloric intake based on sweetness level. By introducing highly sweet products that lack expected calories, we have disrupted this natural control mechanism.

Consider that naturally sweet fruits offer small amounts of fructose balanced with fiber and other protective nutrients that

---

*T. L. Davidson and S. E. Swithers, "A Pavlovian approach to the problem of obesity," *International Journal of Obesity 28* (2004): 933–35.

slow absorption and improve metabolism. The ready availability of manmade sugars that disrupt our natural appetite controls makes it no wonder that obesity rates have skyrocketed.

IMPAIRED IMMUNITY

Sugar is a known immunosuppressant. This is frightening considering that our ability to withstand all diseases, from the common cold to AIDS, depends on having an active, healthy immune system. No matter what form it takes, sugar paralyzes the immune system in a variety of ways:

1. It has been proven to reduce the germ-killing ability of white blood cells for up to five hours after ingestion.

2. It reduces the production of antibodies, proteins that combine with and inactivate foreign invaders in the body.

3. It interferes with the transport of vitamin C, one of the most important nutrients for all facets of immune function.

4. It causes mineral imbalances and sometimes allergic reactions, both of which weaken the immune system.

5. It neutralizes the action of essential fatty acids, thus making cells more permeable to invasion by allergens and microorganisms.

OTHER HEALTH PROBLEMS

All of this should be evidence enough to get the sugar out of your diet, but it's only the tip of the iceberg. Excessive sugar

sugar-related ailments

Acne

Addictions to drugs,
   caffeine, and food

Adrenal gland exhaustion

Alcoholism

Allergies

Anxiety

Appendicitis

Arthritis

Asthma

Behavior problems

Binge eating

Bloating

Bone loss

Cancer (particularly
   breast cancer and
   colon/rectal cancer)

Candidiasis

Cataracts

Colitis

Constipation

Depression

Dermatitis

Diabetes

Difficulty concentrating

Diverticulitis and
   diverticulosis

Eczema

Edema

Emotional problems

Endocrine gland dysfunction

Fatigue

Food cravings

Gallstones

Gout

Heart disease

High blood cholesterol

High estrogen levels

High triglyceride levels

Hormonal problems

Hyperactivity

Hypertension (high blood
   pressure)

Hypoglycemia

Impaired digestion of all
   foods

Indigestion

Insomnia

Kidney stones

Liver dysfunction

Liver enlargement and fatty
   liver syndrome

Low HDL cholesterol

Menstrual difficulties

Mental illness

Mood swings

sugar-related ailments

Muscle pain	Premenstrual syndrome
Nearsightedness	Psoriasis
Obesity	Rheumatism
Osteoporosis	Shortened life span
Overacidity	Tooth decay
Parasitic infections	Ulcers
Premature aging and wrinkles	Vaginal yeast infections
	Weakened immunity

consumption is believed to cause or at least contribute to all of the symptoms, deficiencies, and ailments in the list above. This list was compiled from a detailed review of hundreds of books, articles, and scientific studies that I have researched over the past twenty years.

When I see this list, I find it as overwhelming as you probably do—and I've been looking at the evidence against sugar for more than thirty years! But we have to start believing it. The hard facts are staring us in the face and telling us in no uncertain terms that our health and lives depend upon it.

how much sugar do we need?

Our bodies do not need simple sugars at all.

As amazing as that may sound, here are the facts. The human body needs only about *two teaspoons of sugar* in the bloodstream at any one time. That small amount can easily be obtained through the digestion of complex carbohydrates, protein, and fat. And those complex carbohydrates don't even need to include fruit. We can meet our sugar requirements quite adequately from vegetables, legumes, and grains. (As surprising as that may be, it's true. In fact, some individuals, such as those afflicted with serious yeast infections or those with very high triglyceride levels, need to avoid fruit until their conditions improve. The sugar in fruit feeds yeasts and also raises triglyceride levels just as refined sugar does.)

While most of us do not need to eliminate fruit from our diets, we do need to avoid refined sugar at all costs. As author Nancy Appleton, Ph.D., my colleague and good friend, tells people: "Even if we were to eat no sugar at all, our bodies would still have plenty of sugar. Every teaspoon of refined sugar you eat works to throw the body out of balance and compromise its health."

At this point, you may be saying to yourself, "But I have a sweet tooth. If I shouldn't eat refined sugar, what can I eat to satisfy that sweet tooth?" The answer is simple: fresh fruits and vegetables.

We have to remember that nature provided us with all the sugar we require in vegetables and fruits. These foods also provide the fiber and nutrients we need to properly utilize the sugars they contain. In addition, vegetables and fruits supply powerful, immune-boosting chemicals and antioxidants, some of our best allies to help fight off disease. All of these benefits make vegetables and fruits the only sources of sugars we should regularly include in our daily diets.

The next question you may be asking yourself is "Why does

my body need any sugar?" This answer is not quite as simple. I want to take a moment in this section to explain a subgroup of sugars referred to as "essential sugars" that deserve to be included in your sugar-savvy education. These essential sugars, collectively called *glyconutrients,* build special molecules that coat your cells and act as the communication liaison between cells. So let's briefly review where you can find these essential sugars:

- *Galactose* is found in various vegetables, fruits, and dairy (lactose).
- *Fucose* is found in human breast milk, seaweed, certain medicinal mushrooms, and marine algae.
- *Mannose* is found in blueberries, cranberries, currants, gooseberries, green beans, cabbage, turnips, kelp, and aloe vera.
- *N-acetylgalactosamine* is found in human breast milk and in chondroitin sulfate.
- *N-acetylglucosamine* is found in human breast milk and in glucosamine.
- *N-acetylneuramic acid* is found in human breast milk.
- *Xylose* can be found in xylitol.

As you might imagine, cellular communication plays a crucial role in your system, especially when your body is in crisis. In fact, glyconutrients can help stimulate the immune system when you are sick. It is no wonder that so many of these essential sugars are found in human breast milk. The key here is to remember that these essential sugars are all natural compounds, some made by your body and some found in foods.

so what do we eat?

Once you start realizing how many foods have added sugars and sweeteners, you might ask yourself, "Just what in the world can I eat?"

Before you throw up your hands in despair, let me assure you that you still have plenty of delicious and totally satisfying food options. Low-sugar eating will not leave you wanting as long as you let go of misconceptions about nutrition, such as the claim that all meats and fats are bad for you. Quite to the contrary, protein and essential fatty acids are required to keep your blood sugar balanced. And blood sugar equilibrium, it turns out, is one of the most important but often overlooked keys to health.

We know that too much protein and fat in the diet can cause health problems (just as too little of these nutrients can). We have also learned recently that too many carbohydrates can cause disease. So what's the answer? What constitutes the optimal diet?

The answer is surprisingly simple: *The optimal diet should be balanced.* It should contain sufficient protein from both animal and vegetable sources to help support our bodies' tissue growth and repair, immune integrity, fluid balance, digestive enzyme function, and metabolism. It should contain adequate complex carbohydrates from vegetables, fruits, whole grains, and legumes to give us the best kind of fuel for our muscles and brain functions, and fiber to keep our digestive tracts healthy. And the optimal diet also needs to have sufficient high-quality fat in the form of expeller-pressed oils, nuts, and seeds to help balance blood sugar, strengthen cell and mucous membrane integrity, and provide long-term energy. Ideally, each meal or snack should have an almost equal balance of these three nutrients.

Eating in a balanced way helps promote optimal blood sugar levels. More and more evidence is showing that maintaining balanced blood sugar levels will help you function at your very best. When your blood sugar level is stable, you have extended energy, balanced moods, and greater mental focus and attention. And don't forget that you lessen your risks of developing any of the diseases to which excessive sugar consumption has been linked.

As we know by now, refined sugar should not be a component of the optimal diet. This is becoming glaringly evident. Even the recently developed Food Guide Pyramid warns Americans to limit their sugar consumption.

Since getting sugar out of the diet is vital for good health, your first step must be to get refined sweeteners out of the basic foods you eat every day. This seems almost impossible until you realize that most of the sugars Americans eat come from processed foods. Once you eliminate those sources of hidden sugars and eat natural foods, as your ancestors did, excessive sugar is no longer much of a problem. The guidelines are really pretty simple: Stick to lean meats, fish, eggs, legumes, nuts, whole grains, and vegetables in the entrées and snacks you eat. Once you do this, your diet as a whole becomes low in sugar and you will be able to afford a nutrient-rich sweet treat from time to time without suffering ill effects.

It's natural to have a sweet tooth. After all, the first food we consume—mother's milk—is naturally sweet, and so are fruits and vegetables. The key to satisfying your sweet tooth without experiencing sugar's troublesome health risks is to satisfy it naturally and intelligently. This means turning to moderate amounts of more healthful, nutritious sources of sweets that don't deplete your body as refined sugars do. Getting the sugar out of your diet does not necessarily mean taking the sweetness out. Believe it or not, sweet treats can be a part of a healthy diet as long as you use wholesome ingredients (and a little bit of sugar savvy) in your culinary indulgences.

Whether you decide to enjoy small amounts of natural sweets in moderation, eat them only on rare occasions, or avoid them altogether, this book will help you gain control of the role sugar plays in your life. Doing so will help you enjoy the sweet things in life without the bitter consequences.

using this book

getting the sugar out of your diet involves more than simply passing up dessert. Sugar is pervasive in our society, not only in obvious forms such as cookies, cakes, and candy but also in just about any other food you can think of. From packaged meats to soups to commercial salt, sugar is in there. It's even hidden in such nonfood items as vitamin and mineral supplements, aspirin, prescription and over-the-counter drugs, and various cosmetics.

Cutting down on sugar has to involve a multifaceted approach. It requires developing sugar savvy—knowing where to watch out for sugar and how to creatively and healthfully live without it.

The tips in this book are designed to help you do just that. You probably won't be willing or able to use all 501 suggestions, but that's okay. Remember that this book was written to give helpful hints for everyone: people just wanting to cut refined sugar out of their diets, diabetics who need to cut almost all forms of sugars out, and everyone in between. Just start using the tips that seem easiest and most appealing to you, and your success with those tips may spur you to try others. In any case, even if you incorporate only one-tenth of the tips in this book, you're sure to reduce the sugar in your diet and change your life in a positive and noticeable way.

In addition to avoiding processed sugar, getting the sugar out also means avoiding processed carbohydrate products such as white rice and refined white-flour products such as commercial pasta and bread. These foods are so processed (lacking the fiber and most of the nutrients of the original grain) that they are metabolized just like sugar and almost as fast as sugar.

All of us should try to avoid eating these foods. The evidence is simply too overwhelming that refined carbohydrates such as these cause nutritional deficiencies, wide swings in blood sugar, and degenerative diseases. The more any food is broken down, the more the food's nutrients and fiber are lost—and the more trouble it causes our blood-sugar-regulating mechanisms.

Refined sugar is a perfect example of this. Although the sugar-cane plant has naturally occurring vitamins and minerals, by the time the sugar derived from that plant reaches your sugar bowl, it is essentially a nutrient-void food. In fact, because it supplies you with nothing but empty calories, sugar really acts more like a chemical in the body than a life-giving food. It has been implicated as a causal or contributing factor in some sixty different ailments and diseases, some of which are life-threatening. That's why eliminating refined white sugar is tip number one. It needs to be the top priority in your quest to get the sugar out.

Using natural sweeteners such as the ones mentioned in this book is a relatively easy way to wean yourself from refined sugar, but as you begin replacing sugar with natural sweeteners, remember this: Your ultimate goal should be to reduce the *total* amount of sugars you consume, not simply to exchange white sugar for a more natural sweetener. To help you in this pursuit, I have marked many tips and recipes throughout this book with Sweet Tooth ratings, ranging from 1 to 3. (Tips without a Sweet Tooth rating are simply general concepts you need to understand to develop your sugar savvy, or tips and recipes that satisfy your taste buds in nonsweet ways.)

🦷 **One Sweet Tooth** means that the tips and recipes so marked range from not sweet at all to slightly sweet in nature. Desserts with this rating, for example, will help you satisfy your sweet tooth in a subtle way, which is often all that is needed. Tips with one Sweet Tooth either contain 0 to 4 grams of sugars per serving or rank low on the glycemic index, a scale that measures the rate at which different carbohydrates break down to be released as sugar in the bloodstream. Low-glycemic-index foods release their energy more slowly and steadily and cause less trouble for the body than high-glycemic-index foods.

🦷🦷 **Two Sweet Teeth** are given to those tips, recipes, or foods that provide 5 to 8 grams of sugars per serving and those that contain a combination of foods that together raise your blood sugar level slightly more than low-glycemic-index foods—in other words, foods that produce a moderate blood sugar response. These tips and foods are intermediate ways to indulge your yen for sweetness and can usually be tolerated in moderation when you are in good health and when your diet as a whole is low in sugar.

🦷🦷🦷 **Three Sweet Teeth** are given to those tips and foods that have more than 8 grams of sugars per serving or rank high on the glycemic index. Such foods should only be eaten as rare treats or for special occasions. They can also be used as the means to stop eating white sugar, then eating less sugar altogether. These foods are not low in sugars, but they offer a superior alternative to the usual sweets because they are made with healthful sweeteners instead of white sugar. They will satisfy those who feel the need to have an extra-sweet dessert from time to time, but they should not be eaten often because they can contribute to weight problems, uneven blood sugar levels, and all the other health problems often associated with refined sugar. Foods and recipes designated with Three Sweet Teeth raise the blood sugar very high and very quickly (and can be followed by an equally severe blood sugar "crash") when they aren't balanced with some protein and fat to slow down the release of sugar in the bloodstream. If you have trouble giving up sweets, following Three Sweet Teeth–marked tips is a good place to start and an important step in the right direction, but I wouldn't be honest if I were to tell you that following this step alone will take you far enough to enjoy your best health.

* **Bonus Tips** are also included in this book that are not counted in the 501 tips because they are not specifically about cutting the sugar out of your diet. They will, however, add to your culinary IQ, make things easier in the kitchen, provide valuable nutrition knowledge, or help you toward a new, more interesting way of eating.

Consumer Alerts are special sections of the book that are designed to bring special emphasis to specific areas—the good, the bad, and the ugly.

Throughout *Get the Sugar Out,* I refer to other books, both as sources of recipes and as references for related topics. Since the relationship between sugar and our health is complex, you may want to check out the books in the References section at the end for more detailed information on topics of interest to you.

In addition to references for further reading, I mention specific brand-name products. As long as you pick them with care, convenience products can help you stick to a lower-sugar way of living. The products I have mentioned are not necessarily the only ones or the absolute best ones in a particular category, but they can be very useful. Of course, not every product will agree with you or your lifestyle, so it's up to you to weed out the products (and tips, for that matter) that aren't helpful to you.

Tolerance for sugars and other carbohydrates is an individual thing. Some people may not seem to have a problem metabolizing sugars and refined carbohydrates, while others do. But no matter how well you're handling sugars now, ingesting high-sugar items day after day and year after year will eventually take its toll on your pancreas and adrenal glands.

If you are not currently having health problems on a high-sugar diet, you're fortunate—and unusual. A growing number of Americans—perhaps half of all adults and a larger percentage of the obese—have abused refined sugars and carbohydrates and are developing not only sugar sensitivity but carbohydrate sensitivity as well. More and more research is showing that sugar and carbohydrate sensitivity is associated with such conditions as obesity, heart disease, and diabetes, to name a few.

Therefore, even if you don't presently have health problems, it's much better for you to make gradual changes and cut down on your sugar level now than to wait until later, when your health (and perhaps even your life) might depend on it.

Some of you may have serious conditions that warrant maintenance of extra-strict control over your sugar intake. If you have a weight problem, heart disease, hypoglycemia, diabetes, cancer, yeast problems, parasites, or any condition involving a weak immune system, the evidence is convincing that you should reduce your sugar intake. Individual tolerances do vary, but if you have any of the above conditions, you may even need to avoid natural-sugar-rich fruit until your health improves. I use only natural sweeteners in my diet on occasion because I find I feel better mentally, emotionally, and physically on a very-low-sugar regime. But that's what's right for me.

How far you go in your sugar-slashing quest is entirely up to you. It will depend on your individual biochemistry, your present health, your willpower, and how well you develop your sugar savvy. Make sure to celebrate each of your successful steps toward achieving your long-term goals, no matter how small any given step may seem, and I promise the rewards to your health will be well worth your efforts.

The first reward you get is congratulations from me! By reading this book, you are taking a big step: making a commitment to a healthier way of living. Enjoy yourself as you begin your health-enhancing, sugar-lowering adventure!

get the sugar out of your kitchen

*m*any sugar-cutting tips have multiple uses. Once you learn them, you can use them when making breakfast, lunch, dinner, snacks, and yes, even healthful desserts. They can be utilized time and again until they become habits and maybe even family traditions.

The tips in this chapter are the ones you should begin with. They are fundamental sugar-busters—basic concepts to help you identify sugar in all its various forms and to teach you to limit, substitute for, or eliminate it in the foods you put in your grocery cart, the foods you have in your kitchen, and the way you prepare food.

Start the way that suits you best. Most people like to ease into changes, so begin by remembering the concepts and using the tips that seem the simplest and most appealing to you. Once those become second nature, you'll be more apt to try some of the others.

Lifestyle changes such as cutting the sugar out of your diet have a much better chance of taking root when you know exactly how and why you should make those changes. The tips in this chapter cover those hows and whys and serve as the foundation for all of the other tips in this book. Get to know this chapter well, and remember that the efforts you are putting in today will pay off in rewards to your health tomorrow.

top ten tips

1. **The very easiest way to cut sugar** is to stop adding it to foods such as cereal and fruits and to drinks such as herbal tea, coffee, and coffee substitutes. Simply eliminating nutrient-empty processed sugars from your kitchen is a good way to start. This means not only table sugar but dextrose, raw sugar, turbinado sugar, brown sugar, and powdered sugar as well.

2. **Eliminate processed carbohydrates from your kitchen.** Although many people don't realize it, refined carbohydrates such as white rice, white bread, and white pasta are quickly converted to sugars in the body and disrupt the body's blood sugar and fat control systems. Keeping these common products out of your home is a simple yet effective way to maintain a better-balanced blood sugar level.

3. **Stick with unprocessed whole foods.** That's the only way to be sure you're greatly reducing your sugar intake. Poultry, meat, fish, and eggs are, of course, sugar-free, and legumes, grains, nuts, vegetables, and fruits, which may have some naturally occurring sugars, are full of nutrients and fiber, two ingredients that help balance blood sugar.

4. **Thin out sweeteners or sweet foods,** even natural ones, whenever you can. The idea isn't to substitute one sugar addiction for another one, but rather to gradually and permanently cut down on all forms of sugar in your diet. Dilute concentrated sweeteners such as honey with water and mix sweet foods like granola with unsweet foods such as plain cereal and nuts to reduce the total amount of sugar consumed.

5. **Just as with sugar-free foods, beware of fat-free foods.** The fat-free trend of the early 1990s predated the low-carb craze from which we are now emerging. "Fat-free" may be in bold letters on the label, but what the manufacturers don't tell you is that the products are sugar-rich, sometimes containing two or more times the sugar found in the regular version of that product that naturally contains a little fat. High amounts of sugar not balanced with protein and fat cause the pancreas to release insulin, the body's main fat-storage hormone. Fat-free products may sound good on paper, but in the ultimate irony, fat-free products helped to make Americans fatter and can still do so if you eat them excessively.

6. **The more natural the food, the better.** It's well established now that the more processed a food is, the more it will tend to raise your blood sugar. Since balanced blood sugar levels are the goal, opt for foods as close to their natural state as possible. Choose an orange in place of orange juice, an apple over applesauce, and brown rice instead of white rice.

7. **Become a food detective.** To reduce sugar, you have to know where it is first. To do that, you have to be alert, ask questions, and pay attention to the information you receive about food. Learn to recognize important clues— such as how many grams of sugar are listed on a food label, the ingredients in a food, and how sweet a food tastes to you. Once you identify those foods with a high or hidden sugar content, you know them for what they really are: nutrient robbers and troublemakers for your body.

8. **Eat for taste *and* good nutrition,** not just taste alone. Your tastes can change, after all, but your fundamental nutrient requirements have to be met each and every day. It's far better to have your taste buds rebel for a short while than to have your body break down from nutrient deficiencies. Keep this in mind when you're asked to change long-standing habits for new, healthier, sugar-reducing ways of eating.

9. **Listen to your body.** One of my earlier books, *Your Body Knows Best,* goes into this subject in more depth, but

for now, know that your body gives powerful signals about what's right for you even when your taste buds don't want to listen. For example, if you get an initial high after eating a piece of chocolate but two hours later feel lethargic, irritable, and depressed, your body is going to great lengths to tell you something. Try to pick out those foods that make you feel good over the long term—mentally, emotionally, and physically—and you'll make great strides toward stabilizing your blood sugar.

10. **Eat regular, balanced meals.** This may sound like old-fashioned advice, something your mother might have told you, but scientific research is proving its inherent wisdom. Some research indicates that the body operates more efficiently when each meal or snack that you eat contains approximately 40 percent carbohydrates, 30 percent protein, and 30 percent fat. This formula keeps your blood sugar in the optimal zone for as long as four or five hours. Balanced blood sugar levels mean better concentration, better mood, and greater energy and stamina (and therefore less need or temptation to grab something sweet for quick energy).

tricks of the trade

11. **Try an elimination diet, cutting out sugar in all forms** (even natural sweeteners such as fruit and fruit juice) for

two weeks. This is important as a gauge to help you determine your relationship with sugar. During the two-week period, stick to just poultry, fish, lean meat, whole-grain products, legumes, nuts, and lots of vegetables, and take note of how you feel. If you run into problems, look over the tips in this section and in the "Nutrient Necessities" section in chapter 9.

12. **If you complete the two-week elimination diet** and don't notice any adverse symptoms, try adding a naturally sweetened food back into your diet and see how you respond. If the food doesn't bother you, congratulations! Your sugar metabolism is good; you just need to keep it that way. Use this book to learn creative ways to gradually lower your sugar intake without sacrificing taste so you don't run into blood sugar problems later.

13. **If you can't complete the elimination diet**, don't feel bad. Most Americans have an unhealthy relationship with sugar because they have overindulged in it for so long. Pay special attention to any symptoms you may experience on the elimination diet.

14. **If you experience withdrawal symptoms** such as headaches, moodiness, depression, irritability, and fatigue, you most certainly are addicted to sugar, just as others are addicted to coffee or alcohol. Like alcoholics, who need to avoid alcohol, you also need to eliminate all forms of sugar in your diet, at least until your body chemistry improves.

15. **If you can't go long without eating sugary foods,** you probably have a physical dependence on sugar to give you the quick energy your body is lacking. Switch to eating five or six small, protein-rich meals a day. This will better balance your blood sugar and give you more long-term energy so you're less apt to grab for the sweets.

16. **If eating sugar seems to make all your symptoms go away magically for a short while,** beware. This is often another sign of sugar addiction. Cut out sugars altogether and reduce the amount of other carbohydrates you eat until your body becomes better balanced.

17. **If you lose unwanted weight while eliminating sugar,** congratulations! You will experience firsthand what most people don't realize: *Avoiding sugar is the easiest, safest, and most permanent way to stay slim.* It's a plain and simple fact that too much sugar makes you fat. Use the tips in this book to lower your sugar intake for good and stay trim for life.

18. **If you crave sugar or even complex carbohydrates,** that's almost always a sign that you're not getting enough protein. Emphasize lean meat, poultry, fish, eggs, and properly combined complementary vegetable proteins, and your sugar cravings are likely to diminish.

19. **If you are a vegetarian,** you might want to consider having your amino acid levels tested. Plasma and urine tests often reveal that vegetarians are deficient in the amino acids

lysine, methionine, tryptophan, carnitine, and taurine. Without sufficient amounts of these amino acids, vegetarians can
develop numerous problems, not the least of which are blood
sugar imbalances and sugar and carbohydrate cravings.

20. **When you're under tremendous stress,** the desire for
sweets can be intense. It's worth it to hold your desire at bay,
though. Coping with stress—and maintaining a calm mind
and balanced emotions—surprisingly becomes much, much
easier when you eat well-balanced, nutritious meals and
avoid quick fixes such as alcohol, caffeine, and sugar.

21. **Be sure to get enough sleep.** This is an amazingly simple
prescription, but it can play a huge role in helping you over-
come the sugar blues. When your body is tired, it wants
energy—and that usually translates into sugar binges for
quick fixes. If you give your body the rest it needs, you naturally solve your body's energy problem, and its desire for
sugar will go away as well.

22. **Stock healthful, easy-to-grab, sugar-free foods** for
sudden cravings when you're overworked, tired, or stressed
out. A few good examples are nuts, whole-grain crackers, and
low-fat cheese.

23. **Eat more meals at home,** where you can oversee the ingredients. Restaurants are not above adding sugar to the most
unlikely foods.

24. **Keep sweets out of the house.** If they aren't easily available, you'll be less likely to eat them.

25. **Chew on a cinnamon stick** to help you beat your sweet tooth.

26. **If and when you do eat sugar,** make sure it's with a well-balanced meal or snack. Eating sugar on an empty stomach can cause an initial high followed by a troublesome sugar low. Once your body experiences this sugar low, it will demand more sugar and this up-and-down sugar cycle will continue.

tools of the trade

27. **A blender can help you be a whiz** at whipping up dreamy drinks and desserts with little sugar.

28. **A food processor is an aid as well** when you're using chopped fresh vegetables and fruits in everything from salads to cookies. The fresher your ingredients, the less you'll miss the sugar.

29. **A good set of knives will work also.** It's just that the work required to make your heavenly natural concoctions will take a little more time and muscle. My favorites are from Mac Knife. They combine long-lasting sharpness, effortless slicing, and value with decreased fatigue during use. For more information check out their Web site, www.macknife.com.

30. **A stainless-steel steaming rack** doesn't cost a lot but will pay off in health dividends. Use it to make stuffed, steamed fruits for dessert or steamed organic vegetables that are so delicious on their own they don't need a sugary sauce to enhance their flavor.

31. **Invest in waterless cookware** for a delicious reminder that you don't have to sacrifice taste for health. Without your having to add sugar, salt, fat, or liquid of any kind, food cooks in its own juices and retains vitamins, minerals, other nutrients, essential oils, texture, and flavor. Plus, these chock-full-of-goodness foods may actually decrease your appetite since your body feels satisfied because it is getting what it needs from your cooking as opposed to cooking off all of these essential ingredients into the water. To cook the tastiest and easiest sugar-free foods you've ever tasted, treat yourself to Saladmaster's Versa Tec Health System. Check it out at www.healthsourcesystems.com/versa.htm.

32. **A wide-mouth thermos is a good purchase** that will come in handy for taking homemade sugar-free soups, stews, and leftovers wherever you go. Or use it to carry sugar-free hot herbal teas or grain-based coffee substitutes.

33. **Use measuring spoons and cups to be precise** about the amount of sweetener you add while cooking. An extra tablespoon of honey might not seem like much, but it adds an extra *18 grams of sugars* to your dish. (That's 72 more calories!)

tasteful techniques

34. **Learn to enjoy the taste of foods as they are** without any added sugar. This may take a little time, particularly if you're currently a sugarholic, but your taste buds will change. If you stick with a low-sugar diet, in time not only won't you like the taste of the sickeningly sweet foods you used to indulge in, but you'll appreciate the subtle but terrific tastes of simply prepared foods.

35. **Explore the five tastes.** There's more to life than sweetness, you know! In fact, in the ancient five-element theory of food therapy in Chinese medicine, it's taught that too much of one taste can cause imbalance in the body. Most Americans have a love affair with both the sweet taste and the salty taste and don't experience the pleasure that the other tastes can bring: bitter (as in mustard greens), sour (as in a lemon), and pungent (as in a radish).

36. **Cut down on salt to lessen your cravings for sugar.** This may sound far-fetched, but it's a tip the Chinese knew about more than five thousand years ago. According to Oriental philosophy, salty foods cause a contraction or tightening of the body's fluids and tissues, while sweet foods do the exact opposite: They cause the body to expand or relax. If you overindulge in salty foods, your body usually craves sweet foods as a way to maintain balance. By cutting down on one, you'll automatically start cutting down on the other. The next time you crave sweets, ask yourself, "Have I been eating too much salt?"

• •

37. **Our sense of taste is intimately connected with our sense of smell,** a little-mentioned but important piece of information that you can use to increase your enjoyment of subtly sweetened foods. By using fresh, aromatic herbs, spices, and natural extracts, your nose will love the smell of the sugar-reduced foods you eat and your taste buds will perceive the foods as sweeter than they really are.

38. **Develop a fear of commercial desserts,** which not only are sweetened with entirely too much sugar but also commonly contain white flour, questionable preservatives, and harmful trans fats (in the form of margarine, shortening, rancid oils, and hydrogenated or partially hydrogenated oils).

39. **Satisfy your sweet tooth naturally** with fresh fruit or desserts made with natural ingredients. These treats give you vitamins, minerals, and fiber that lifeless desserts made with white flour and white sugar simply don't provide.

40. **A treat doesn't have to be sweet.** Sometimes it just has to be something new and different, something that breaks up your usual routine. As you begin cutting the sugar out, start exploring interesting, nutritious foods that have recently been rediscovered or become commercially available. This book discusses many such foods. Don't be afraid to try them.

spicing life

41. **Experiment with spices and herbs,** nature's gifts of flavor to us. Your taste buds might become so intrigued by the flavorful tastes of various herbs and spices such as caraway, sage, and cayenne that you simply no longer need so many sweet tastes to satisfy them.

42. **Coriander, nutmeg, ginger, and cardamom** are all spices that can make a dish taste sweeter and help satisfy your sweet tooth without adding any sugar.

43. **Natural vanilla extract and cinnamon are classics** when it comes to upping your perceived level of sweetness. If you don't believe that, try this taste test, passed on to me by cookbook author and health-spa menu consultant Jeanne Jones: Pour 1 cup milk and add 1 teaspoon vanilla extract and ¼ teaspoon cinnamon. Mix thoroughly, then ask someone to taste it and tell you what you put in it. The answer will almost always be "sugar." Use this common perception to increase your enjoyment of everything from cereal and milk to sugar-free sweet treats.

44. **Other natural flavoring extracts** open up a world of taste possibilities without any extra sugar. Test your imagination by using almond, mint, coconut, or lemon extracts and see how once-boring foods are suddenly transformed into new taste sensations. Look for Spicery Shoppe, Frontier Herbs, and other brands that use natural ingredients in their extracts

instead of artificial ones. Artificial colors and flavors are made from coal-tar derivatives and definitely don't have a place in a healthy diet.

45. **Cinnamon, cloves, and bay leaves** might soon be just what the doctor orders to help regulate blood sugar levels. Test-tube studies conducted at the U.S. Department of Agriculture's Vitamin and Mineral Laboratory have shown that these spices triple insulin's ability to metabolize sugar and remove it from the blood. To give your body extra help maintaining blood sugar balance, add these spices to foods and drinks whenever possible.

46. **Crush dried herbs and spices with a mortar and pestle** before adding them to a dish. Doing so will release the spices' aroma and dramatically increase the food's flavor.

47. **Learn the art of infusion** and add a gourmet flair to an everyday oil. Simply soak fresh herbs in a bottle of expeller-pressed oil and season salads or vegetables without any sugar.

those "sugarless" sugars

48. **Giving up sugar is hard,** but don't be tempted to use an artificial sweetener as an alternative. This may seem like an easy way out, but you may be surprised to learn that an artificial sweetener doesn't really offer any of its advertised advantages and can cause you plenty of harm, as this section will explain.

49. **The use of artificial sweeteners hasn't diminished Americans' sugar intake;** it actually seems to have given users more of a sweet tooth! The fact is that since artificial sweeteners came into wide use, about thirty years ago, total consumption of sweeteners has substantially increased. A number of studies have shown that ingestion of artificial sweeteners may actually lead to increased food or calorie intake. This is likely because artificial sweeteners cause your body to produce insulin by making it think sugar is on the way.

50. **Artificial sweeteners haven't helped with weight loss either.** Roughly 65 percent of the American public is now overweight even though the consumption of artificial sweeteners has skyrocketed in the last decade.

51. **Aspartame (known as Equal or NutraSweet)** may deplete the body's supplies of chromium, a trace mineral known to play a crucial role in sugar metabolism. Insufficient chromium leads to insulin inefficiency, which, in turn, leads to greater insulin resistance or carbohydrate intolerance. (For more information check out **"Consumer Alert: What You Need to Know About the Top Two Artificial Sugar Substitutes"** on page 55.)

52. **Splenda, NutraSweet, Equal, and Sweet'n Low all are sources of "hidden" sugar.** Believe it or not, even though these sweeteners are advertised as ways to avoid it, sugar—in the form of dextrose—is in the ingredient list of each of them.

53. The use of aspartame can increase sugar and carbohydrate cravings. This is because phenylalanine, one of aspartame's components, blocks production of serotonin, a neurotransmitter that sends messages from the pineal gland in the brain. When the body's production of serotonin is out of order, a multitude of symptoms, ranging from premenstrual syndrome to depression, can result. Most important, insufficient serotonin causes more sugar and carbohydrate cravings and increases the likelihood of binge eating.

* *Bonus Tip* Neotame is another aspartame look-alike that has made its debut. The FDA approved it for general use in July 2002 and states that it is safe for children, pregnant and lactating women, and people with diabetes. In fact, this product was developed to fill a medical market gap that aspartame doesn't cover. Since people suffering from phenylketonuria (PKU) cannot safely use aspartame, NutraSweet manufacturers developed Neotame. Neotame does not metabolize into phenylalanine (as aspartame does), so it is considered safe for this group.

54. More than 75 percent of all nondrug complaints to the Food and Drug Administration concerned aspartame up until the FDA stopped recording aspartame-specific complaints. Aspartame sensitivity or overload can reveal itself through symptoms such as headaches, blurred vision, anxiety

consumer alert
WHAT YOU NEED TO KNOW ABOUT THE TOP TWO ARTIFICIAL SUGAR SUBSTITUTES

ASPARTAME (aka NutraSweet, Equal, Canderel) is 160–200 times as sweet as sugar.

Note: Another similar compound that is also made from amino acids, alitame, is now seeking a place in your local store.

• In 1965 James M. Schlatter synthesized aspartame while producing an antiulcer drug candidate. In fact, the compound was considered as a potential sweetener only after Schlatter happened to lick his finger, which had accidentally been contaminated with the compound.

• When ingested, aspartame breaks down into several constituent chemicals, including aspartic acid, phenylalanine, methanol, and further breakdown products including formaldehyde and formic acid.

• It is unstable under heat and changing pH conditions.

• Initial safety testing suggested that this caused brain tumors in rats.

• In 1980 the FDA's Public Board of Inquiry (PBOI) recommended against approving aspartame at that time, citing "unanswered questions about cancer in laboratory rats."

• In 1981 newly appointed FDA commissioner Arthur Hull Hayes, citing data from a Japanese study that had not been available to the PBOI, approved aspartame for use in dry foods.

(continued)

Hayes had confirmed ties with the artificial sweetener industry; most notably, he was close friends with Donald Rumsfeld, at the time CEO of the company that manufactured NutraSweet (aspartame).

• In 1983 the FDA approved aspartame for use in carbonated beverages, other beverages, baked goods, and confections.

• In 1995, the FDA Epidemiology Branch chief reported that aspartame complaints represented 75 percent of all reports of adverse reactions to substances in the food supply from 1981 to 1995. Consumers and physicians reported approximately ninety-two different symptoms and health conditions.

• In 1996 the FDA removed all restrictions on use.

• Individuals with the previously mentioned condition PKU should not consume this product.

• Aspartame is available in approximately 6,000 consumer foods and beverages sold worldwide.

SUCRALOSE (aka Splenda) is 600 times as sweet as table sugar. It has overtaken Equal as the most popular artificial sweetener.

• It was discovered in 1976. Put simply, it is made by *chlorinating* sugar! Yes, its manufacture involves the same chemical found in swimming pools. How could this be? It was discovered through a misunderstanding. Two Tate & Lyle scientists were looking for a way to test chlorinated sugars as chemical intermediates when there was a gross misunderstanding. Leslie Hough asked his young Indian colleague

Shashikant Phadnis to test the powder. Phadnis thought Hough said "taste," and he did—it was very sweet! A final sweetener formula was developed within a year.

• Sucralose is composed of 50 percent phenylalanine, 40 percent aspartic acid, and 10 percent methyl alcohol.

• Sucralose mixed with maltodextrin and dextrose (both made from corn) as bulking agents is sold internationally as Splenda.

• In 1998 it was approved by the U.S. FDA; as of 2006 it has been approved in more than sixty countries.

• In 2000 concerns over safety surfaced, including lack of long-term studies.

• Whole Foods Market took an official stand that it will not carry any products containing sucralose because, as the company points out, most of the studies were commissioned by organizations that had a financial interest in the approval of sucralose.

• Reported symptoms of sensitivity to this compound include headaches, dizziness/balance problems, mood swings, vomiting and nausea, abdominal pain and cramps, seizures and convulsions, and changes in vision. Concerns have also been raised regarding its effect on the thymus gland, crucial to proper immune system functioning.

• Sucralose can be found in more than 4,500 food and beverage products.

• Marketed in the United States as a "no-calorie sweetener," Splenda does contain 96 calories a cup, approximately eight times fewer than sugar by volume.

attacks, seizures, menstrual cramps, mood swings, loss of energy, and heart-attack-like symptoms. If you feel you may be affected, eliminate use and become a better food detective.

55. Using saccharin, another artificial sweetener known most often under the brand name Sweet'n Low, has its own set of risks. Saccharin is a petroleum derivative that may be harmful to sensitive individuals. For this reason, it has been banned in foods in such countries as Germany and France for almost a century. The brand names for saccharin are Necta Sweet, Sweet'n Low, Sweet'n Low Brown, and Sweet Twin. These are 200–700 times sweeter than good old sucrose or white sugar. Saccharin can be found in gum, cosmetics, and prescription drugs.

56. New versions of sugar alcohols may satisfy a sweet tooth but leave your stomach in knots. Mannitol, sorbitol, and hydrogenated starch hydrolysate are some of the new kids on the block. These noncaloric sweeteners are laxatives and, when taken frequently or in large doses, often cause uncomfortable gastrointestinal bloating, cramps, and diarrhea. Common ingredients in sugar-free chewing gums, sorbitol and mannitol do not promote cavities in the mouth, but they have been shown to nourish and increase the number of *Streptococcus mutans* bacteria, which do cause cavities. Zsweet is a patent-pending blend of erythritol and natural flavor enhancers that is made by fermentation and is slightly sweeter than table sugar. It claims to be better tolerated with higher digestibility.

✳ ***Bonus Tip*** Malitol is one of the more recent sugar alcohols used as a sugar substitute in sugarless hard candies, chewing gum, ice cream, chocolates, and baked goods. It is a hydrogenation of maltose, obtained from starch, and is sold under the names Maltisorb and Maltisweet. It has roughly 90 percent of the sweetness of table sugar and does not brown or carmelize like the white stuff. While it may have few calories, less effect on blood sugar, and less potential for tooth decay than table sugar, it does come with one significant and recognized downside—gastric distress (especially in larger quantities).

✳ ***Bonus Tip* #2** Of all the sugar alcohols, xylitol, also called wood sugar or birch sugar, is a natural standout. It is a five-carbon compound that is naturally found in the fibers of many fruits and vegetables as well as corn fiber and birch trees. Commercially available since the 1960s, it not only contains 40 percent fewer calories than sugar, but it inhibits oral bacteria and helps prevent plaque and cavities. Not surprisingly, it was first introduced in chewing gums. Six international dental associations have even officially endorsed xylitol. Studies have shown that its natural chemical structure combined with the act of chewing can prevent ear infections. Animal studies suggest that it may also prevent weakening of the bones and improved bone density. On the downside, xylitol may cause potentially fatal liver toxicity in dogs. Xylitol Pure is Jarrow Formula's brand of all-natural xylitol crystals for one-to-one substitution with

(continued)

ordinary sugar; it is available through the Web site www. jarrow.com. Xylitol Unique Gum and Mints come in a wide assortment of flavors, are made only with xylitol, and are available through the Web site www.vrp.com.

If you are already aware of xylitol but have noticed that from time to time it is not always easily available, your observations are correct. In fact, in 2007 there may have been a very real shortage of xylitol on the market. Rumor has it that a big factor in this shortage was a xylitol-producing plant shutdown. The factory was being refitted for expansion in order to be able to meet increasing demand for xylitol in food and beverage formulations in both Europe and Japan. Due to this shortage, the company that makes xylitol began offering an alternative, erythritol. One company I suggest you check out is at www.xylitol.com, and features a new PolySweet High-Grade Erythritol. This site claims that, "unlike xylitol, it has little to no laxative effect in higher amounts (better tolerated), near zero calories, and mixes better in low-calorie beverages, candies, and chocolates."

* *Bonus Tip #3* Erythritol sounds quite promising indeed. In fact, in many circles it is being hailed as the new best sugar substitute. It bears repeating once again that, unlike other sugar alcohols, erythritol does not cause stomach distress. It is produced by a natural fermentation process of easily available glucose from ingredients such as corn, potatoes, rice, or any other food source that contains sugars or complex carbohydrates. This makes it easier (and cheaper) and even more "healthy" to produce than most of its coun-terparts, including xylitol, which can be relatively expensive and is derived mainly from birchwood fibers that have been subjected to unnatural acids, chemical catalysts, and high pressures and temperatures in a series of separation and purification techniques. While there are some newer and more natural fermentation techniques for producing xylitol on the horizon, erythritol seems poised to step into the sugar substitute spotlight.

The top four reasons to use erythritol would be that it is safe for diabetics, it does not promote tooth decay, it is 70 percent as sweet as sucrose with only 0.2 calories per gram, and it can help maintain healthy colonic pH and ecol-ogy, as opposed to creating discomfort and gas like many other sugar alcohols. You can find a tabletop version of this sweetener as Smart Sweet Granules Organic Erythritol at www.globalsweet.com or by calling 800-601-0688.

57. **Acesulfame potassium** is commercially sold under the brand names Sunette, Sweet & Safe, and Sweet One. This substance is 200 times sweeter than sucrose. The Center for Science in the Public Interest has studied the safety issues regarding this sweetener and has concluded that acesulfame potassium probably causes cancer. Add this to the list of sweeteners to avoid.

58. **The best way to kick the sugar habit** is to use the sug-gestions in this book and not to turn to artificial sweeteners,

no matter what form they take. The human body simply wasn't designed to deal with these unnatural chemicals. Using them is likely to cause different but equally severe or perhaps more harmful problems than those that sugar causes.

sweeteners worth noting

59. **Dehydrated cane juice crystals,** sold under the commercial name Sucanat, are the easiest sweetening substitute for people who are used to white sugar. Made by evaporating the water from sugarcane juice, Sucanat contains the nutrients that naturally occur in sugarcane. It can be used in the same amount as the sugar required in a recipe, but be careful with it: Most recipes use entirely too much sugar, and even in small amounts, Sucanat can cause adverse symptoms in anyone who is allergic to cane sugar.

60. **Maple syrup** is a natural sweetener best used in small amounts. Made by boiling down maple sap, maple syrup contains a full complement of minerals and is particularly rich in potassium and calcium. Another sweetener, maple sugar, is made when maple syrup is dehydrated. (See tip 88 for additional information.)

61. **Honey** is a natural sweetener because it is made by bees, but it is sweeter, has more calories, and raises the blood sugar even more than white sugar. However, truly natural honey has some reported medicinal benefits and contains enzymes

and small amounts of minerals, so it does not upset the body's mineral balance as much as refined sugar. In addition, baked goods made with honey have the added benefit of remaining fresher longer than those made with other sweeteners. And if you have blood sugar issues, remember that honey is still sugar. (See tip 88.) Two good brands to try are Really Raw Honey, www.reallyrawhoney.com, and Tropical Traditions, www.tropicaltraditions.com.

✳ *Bonus Tip* Never give an infant under eighteen months of age honey or products made with honey. This sweetener sometimes contains trace amounts of botulinum spores, which are easily rendered harmless by the mature digestive tract of an adult but can be harmful or even fatal to an infant, whose digestive tract is just developing.

✳ *Bonus Tip #2* Manuka honey is an especially potent honey rich in phytonutrients that are very aggressive against the *E. coli* and *H. pylori* superbugs. It is known as "nature's sweetest bacteria-buster" and can be ordered at www.wedderspoon.com and www.manukahoneyusa.com.

62. **Blackstrap molasses** is the residue after crystals of sugar are removed from beet juice or sugarcane. Although it still contains 65 percent sucrose, blackstrap molasses contains measurable amounts of minerals, especially calcium and iron, making it more nutritious than most other sweeteners. Other

types of molasses, such as sorghum molasses and Barbados molasses, are made in a similar process but are much less nutritious than the blackstrap variety.

* **Bonus Tip** One of the many urban legends behind the long use of blackstrap molasses is that it can reverse the graying of hair. While there is no real scientific evidence to support this, the biochemistry of this sweetener might make you think otherwise. Consider that gray hair is thought to be caused by a deficiency in copper and B vitamins. Blackstrap molasses is very high in copper as well as iron, B vitamins, calcium, and potassium.

63. **Agave syrup or nectar** is made from the fruit of the agave, a cactus-like plant native to Mexico. It ranks low on the glycemic index yet is roughly 75 percent sweeter than sugar and can be used to sweeten just about any type of food or drink.

* **Bonus Tip** Aguamiel, a similar though less popular alternative, is a thick, dark, distinctive-tasting sweetener made from maguey cactus plants. With a taste somewhat reminiscent of molasses, aguamiel is best used in small amounts for sweetening bean recipes. If you are interested in trying aguamiel, ask your local health food store to order it for you.

64. **Amasake (from rice), rice syrup, barley malt, and sorghum syrup** are sweeteners prepared by fermenting the grains from which they came. The fermenting bacteria convert many of the grains' starches into simple sugars and also some complex sugars. In addition, these grain-based liquid sweeteners contain some of the nutrients that are found in the whole grains.

65. **Try rice syrup powder and milk sugar,** two natural sweeteners from foods you don't necessarily think of as sweet. Rice syrup powder, sold commercially as DevanSweet, is half as sweet as sugar but can be substituted for it in equal amounts to create a less sweet version of a recipe. Made from evaporated rice syrup, it also contains some minerals and complex carbohydrates, as rice syrup does. Tagatose is a natural sweetener (sold as Shugr, Sweet Fiber, and TheraSweet) that is made from milk sugar (lactose). It has one-third the calories of table sugar and is nearly 92 percent as sweet, plus it doesn't raise blood sugar. It is recognized by the FDA as a safe additive and is available in tabletop form; however, it may cause flatulence, especially in lactose-intolerant people.

66. **Fruit and dried fruit** are, of course, one of the best options for sweetening foods. Mashed banana, chopped apple, and raisins are just some of the ways to naturally satisfy your sweet tooth and get a healthy dose of vitamins and minerals. Remember, though, that while a little fruit may be healthy, too much fruit can cause all the problems that sugar can cause.

67. **Date "sugar"** is made from pulverized dried dates. It has the consistency of sugar but isn't refined like sugar. It also contains fiber and is high in many minerals. In addition, since date "sugar" is just dried fruit, it is allowed on sugar-restricted diets. One tablespoon of date "sugar" is counted as one fruit exchange in the diabetic exchange system, a listing of food portions from each food group in which each portion is interchangeable with others in the same group. Look for this sweetener in natural food stores.

68. **Fruit juice and fruit juice concentrates,** common ingredients in goodies sold in health food stores, are concentrated sources of sugar that contain the nutrients present in fresh fruit but none of the fiber that balances blood sugar. These sweeteners can quickly flood your bloodstream with sugar, then cause an equally fast fall in blood sugar if they are not balanced with some protein, fat, and fiber. When making your own baked goods or desserts, try to use fruit juice

> * ***Bonus Tip*** Besides giving you all of the sugar from pounds and pounds of fruit, commercial fruit juice and juice concentrates also unfortunately become concentrated sources of the fungicides and pesticides used on all that fruit. For this reason, be sure to go out of your way to buy organic varieties. There's no sense making a goodie full of nutritious ingredients and then ruining it by adding a sweetener full of harmful chemicals.

consumer alert
NOT ALL JUICES ARE CREATED EQUAL

Two-thirds of the HFCS consumed in the United States is in beverages. While soft drinks top the list in this area, juices and flavored drinks have increasingly added this cheap, readily available sweetener. Since such a large part of the juice market has fallen victim to HFCS (and labels can be confusing and deceiving), I wanted to call special attention to a few juices that deserve a place in your grocery cart.

• **Noni juice** may act as an antiwrinkle agent as well as an anti-inflammatory, anticancer agent, and antioxidant. Sadly, its taste in pure form (the best form) is not the greatest, so small servings are recommended.

• **Goji berries** are another example of how good things come in small packages. They contain eighteen amino acids and up to twenty-one trace minerals, as well as carotenoids, vitamin C, and natural fiber.

• **Welch's Guava Pineapple Juice** comes from South America and is loaded with vitamin C (250 percent of your RDA per serving) and lycopene for heart health.

• **Bolthouse Farms Passion Fruit Apple Carrot Juice** comes from New Zealand and the United States and is loaded with lycopene as well as cancer-fighting polyphenols.

• **Mountain Sun Grape & Acai** is from the Amazon basin and is loaded with cholesterol fighters, including anthocyanins, flavonoids with extremely high antioxidant activity

(continued)

(four times more than red grapes) as well as the ability to fight inflammation. Plus it can help protect blood vessels and the nervous system (including the brain).

• **Adina Pömagic Pomegranate Mangosteen** is from Southeast Asia and is loaded with xanthones, which may reduce inflammation and decrease the risk of heart disease.

instead of juice concentrates or fruit syrups, which are even more condensed, and be sure to use any juice sweetener judiciously.

69. **Fructose** is a natural sugar found in fruit that as a commercial sweetener is usually made from corn and is, of course, related to high-fructose corn syrup (but is not as deleterious to health). A highly refined product, like sugar, it is devoid of nutrients but is included in this book because it scores low (only 20) on the glycemic index. In other words, it stimulates insulin secretion only slightly, causing less of a rise and fall in blood sugar levels; this means it can be tolerated by *some* hypoglycemics and diabetics. Fructose is sweeter than sucrose, so less is needed to obtain the same sweetness in a recipe. As with all sweeteners, use fructose in small amounts if you can tolerate it. Large amounts have been shown to increase artery-clogging LDL cholesterol levels, raise uric acid levels in the blood, and cause diarrhea and gastrointestinal pain in some people. It is also known to raise

triglyceride levels more than any other type of sugar. (See tip 87.)

70. **Stevia** is a sweet herb that is the sweetener of choice for many afflicted with conditions such as candidiasis and parasites. It has been used for hundreds of years as a sweetener in South America and now has wide commercial value in Japan, where it is put in everything from soft drinks to soy sauce. Stevia has thirty times the sweetness of sugar and negligible calories, and it does not raise blood sugar like other caloric sweeteners. The FDA has approved its use as a food supplement but not as a food additive. Since 1 teaspoon of stevia powder has the sweetening power of 2 to 4 cups of sugar, the most common way to use stevia is to make a liquid concentrate with it (using 1 teaspoon powder mixed in 3 tablespoons water) and add a drop or two to sweeten drinks and foods.

71. **Fructooligosaccharides (FOS)** are sucrose molecules to which one, two, or three additional fructose molecules have been attached. Naturally occurring in fruits, and some grains and vegetables, FOS provide your taste buds with the taste of sugar, but the molecules are too big to be digested by the body as sugar. Since FOS aren't digested, this sweetener doesn't affect blood sugar levels. It also can't be utilized by *Candida albicans*, other yeasts, and some bacteria. The best news about FOS, though, is that it provides a benefit that none of the other sweeteners do: It nourishes and promotes the growth of friendly intestinal bacteria such as bifidobacteria in

your large intestine without feeding pathogenic bacteria. This makes it a potential good-for-you sweetener for people struggling with yeast infections, parasites, and other gastrointestinal disorders. The Japanese have been using FOS for several decades with no adverse effects reported, though in large doses it may cause soft stools or diarrhea. The product Stevia Plus, available in health food stores throughout the country, contains FOS in its Frutafit Inulin Fiber. The product Flora-Key, distributed by Uni Key Health Systems (www.unikeyhealth.com), also contains FOS as part of its formula. With Flora-Key you get the best of both worlds: a probiotic that is supported and fed by a prebiotic.

72. **Determine which natural sweeteners are best for you.** One person may feel best using fructose, while another may tolerate honey better. Since our individual body chem-

---

✳ *Bonus Tip*   There is a terrific new sweetener on the market known as SweetPerfection. This new sweetener is an ultra-low-glycemic-index sweetener that can be used like sugar in tea, coffee, and baking. SweetPerfection is naturally high in fiber. It is chicory root ground to a powder that is very high in soluble fiber and looks and tastes exactly like sugar. It has an ultra-low glycemic index, approximately zero; it will not cause insulin surges and it is 100 percent guaranteed to taste and perform exactly like sugar. Check it out at www.lowcarbspecialties.com.

istries are so different, the foods we each feel best eating will vary as well.

73. **Use the least concentrated, least sweet, and smallest amounts** of sweeteners possible. Remember that a sugar is still sugar to the body, no matter how natural it may be.

---

supermarket savvy

74. **Concentrate your grocery shopping in the outer aisles.** Foods on the inner aisles are designed to have a long shelf life, and sugar is one of the most common preservatives for this purpose. Shop the outer aisles—the produce, meat, dairy, and bulk foods sections—and take some of the guesswork out of what to buy. It's by far the best way to shop.

75. **Become a label reader.** There's just no way around it: If you're going to buy packaged foods, you have to pay attention to what's in them. Three-quarters of the sugars Americans ingest are hidden in processed foods, so you have to become skeptical about every food you're thinking of buying. Read those labels, educate yourself, and don't let the hidden sugar slip past you.

76. **Label-Reading Lesson #1:** Read the number of sugar grams listed on the Nutrition Facts label of the food you're considering buying. The lower the number of sugar grams, the

better off you are. As a general guideline, look for foods that contain 3 grams of sugars or less per serving.

77. **If it helps you to understand grams of sugars in terms of teaspoons of sugar,** realize that there are 4 grams of sugars in every teaspoon (or packet) of sugar. A can of soda that has 40 grams of sugar, therefore, is the equivalent of having a can of sparkling water with flavoring, then adding 10 teaspoons of sugar to it.

78. **Label-Reading Lesson #2:** Compare the number of sugar grams to the number of total carbohydrate grams. Avoid foods that have more than one-third of their total carbohydrates coming from sugars. The majority of the carbohydrates you consume each day should be of the complex variety, not from simple sugars. To help you eat this way, shop for foods with the lowest number of sugar grams in relation to their carbohydrate grams.

79. **Label-Reading Lesson #3:** Peruse the ingredients list and look for sugar in all its various forms. It can be listed as any of the following: barley malt, beet sugar, brown sugar, buttered syrup, cane-juice crystals, cane sugar, caramel, carob syrup, corn syrup, corn syrup solids, date sugar, dextran, dextrose, diastase, diastatic malt, ethyl maltol, fructose, fruit juice, fruit juice concentrate, glucose, glucose solids, golden sugar, golden syrup, grape sugar, high-fructose corn syrup, honey, invert sugar, lactose, malt syrup, maltodextrin, maltose, mannitol, molasses, raw sugar, refiner's syrup, sor-

bitol, sorghum syrup, sucrose, sugar, turbinado sugar, and yellow sugar. These are all ingredients you want to be mindful of.

80. **Label-Reading Lesson #3 (Short Version):** A quick way to discern sugars on the label is simply to look for the word *sugar* in any form and for words ending in *-ose*.

> ✳ ***Bonus Tip*** While you're reading the label for sugar content, pay attention to the other ingredients in the food as well. If there are ingredients that you can't pronounce or spell, much less recognize, the chances are good that the product belongs more in a laboratory experiment than in your body. Skip the fake foods and instead buy products that have identifiable whole foods as ingredients.

81. **Label-Reading Lesson #4:** Pay attention if a label lists how many fruit exchanges in the diabetic food-exchange system the food counts as. In my experience counseling clients, I have found that even healthy individuals usually do better when they limit themselves to two to four fruit exchanges per day. Even if you aren't diabetic, choose products that count as one fruit exchange or less to avoid overconsumption of even natural-sugar-rich, fruit-sweetened foods.

82. **Understand the meaning of "sugar-free"** under the FDA's food-labeling rules. It means that the food contains less than 0.5 grams of sugar per serving (a great goal to shoot for).

> ✻ *Bonus Tip* Be careful of foods with old labels on them or cookbooks that mention they are "sugar-free." Many labels and older cookbooks were printed before the new labeling requirements went into effect, and the foods and recipes in them definitely don't qualify as "sugar-free."

83. **"No added sugar," "without added sugar," and "no sugar added"** are recently regulated terms that mean that no sugar or ingredients containing sugars (e.g., fruit juices, applesauce, or dried fruit) were added during the processing

> ✻ *Bonus Tip* "Sugar-free" and "no added sugar" signal a reduction in calories from sugars only, not from fat, protein, and other carbohydrates. If the total calories are not reduced, a statement will appear next to the "sugar-free" claim explaining that the food is "not low-calorie" or "not for weight control." If the total calories are reduced, the "sugar-free" claim must be accompanied by a "low-calorie" or "reduced-calorie" claim.

or packing of the product and that the product has no ingredients that were made with added sugars, such as jams, jellies, or concentrated fruit juices.

84. **A "reduced-sugar" product** contains at least 25 percent less sugar than the original product.

85. **Don't be fooled** by manufacturers looking to capitalize on consumers' desire to buy natural sugars. Although they may sound or look healthier than white sugar, all of the following are fancy terms for refined sugars that give you nothing but empty calories: blond sugar, brown sugar, natural sugar, raw sugar, turbinado sugar, and yellow-D sugar.

86. **While all-natural is almost always the way to go when it comes to choosing food,** the term "all-natural" on a label doesn't have any real meaning and certainly doesn't mean that the product is low in sugars. An increasing number of sweeteners—brands such as FruitSource, for example—are made from all-natural ingredients but are highly concentrated sources of sugars. Use them by the pinch or by the drop if you must, but by all means, do not use them with abandon.

87. **If fructose is your sweetener of choice,** you should probably curtail both pure crystalline fructose as well as the liquid variety. Liquid fructose is actually isomerized corn syrup.

88. **Be careful to buy 100 percent pure maple syrup and honey.** If you grab the wrong stuff because it's priced below all the others or because you're in a hurry, you could be buying a mixture of mostly corn syrup instead. One thing to look for in your search for nutrient-dense honey is the hardness or literal density of the product, because hardness indicates the level of live-state nutrients and heat-sensitive enzymes. That said, pasteurization and high-heat processing (over 105 degrees) destroys many of the beneficial enzymes and phyto-nutrients.

89. **Don't go grocery shopping when you're hungry.** If your stomach is empty as you browse the aisles, your plummeting blood sugar will tempt you to buy high-sugar items instead of nutritional staples. Eat a well-rounded meal before you go shopping to avoid coming home with bags full of junk food.

the fine art of moderation

90. **Eat a sweet treat slowly, one small forkful at a time, and savor it.** When you allow yourself to get pure enjoyment from your indulgence, you'll be satisfied with a small amount and won't want to eat the whole thing.

91. **Better yet, split it.** Your friend or lover will adore you for sharing your dessert, and your body will be happier with the arrangement as well.

92. **Do not restrict yourself to the point of causing a sugar binge.** Human nature is such that we always seem to yearn for the things we can't have. Giving yourself a touch of sweetness here and there may be a better strategy in the long run than total abstinence.

93. **Try limiting your sugar intake for six days at a time** and then, on the seventh day, allow yourself to eat a serving of any sweet treat you want. This tip helps to instill moderation in those who tend to have an all-or-nothing attitude toward sugar.

94. **Another moderation strategy is this:** Allow yourself indulgences during vacations or special occasions, but once your regular routine begins again, go back to your low-sugar diet for life. One male friend of mine has made this practice into a real science, being able to maintain his weight despite his occasional culinary "splurges."

95. **Do the best you can at reducing your sugar intake,** but don't be too hard on yourself. Remember that if you aren't always perfect, it's because you're a human being, not a robot. If you ate more sweets today than you would have liked, accept it and just vow to eat better tomorrow. Mistakes can be helpful if you use them as lessons.

96. **Avoiding sweets is important for good health,** but just as important is a healthy attitude and a balanced lifestyle. Your desire to cut down on sugar is commendable, but be sure to

keep it in perspective with other factors that contribute to a healthy quality of life: avoidance of damaged fats, unnecessary chemicals, and environmental toxins; regular exercise; a positive self-image; and meaningful work and personal relationships.

get the sugar out
of breakfast

*m*ost people would never think of trying to start their car in the morning without any fuel or with the wrong type of fuel. They know that the car most likely wouldn't run, or if it did, it certainly wouldn't run efficiently.

But many Americans don't have the same respect for their bodies as they do for their cars. They start their day with coffee and a Danish, an instant breakfast shake and a Pop-Tart, or a sugar-laden, fat-free muffin—then wonder why they don't have any energy two hours later. Some even leave the house for a full day of work with nothing in their stomachs at all, yet they are dismayed when they don't experience their optimal level of mental, emotional, and physical functioning later in the day.

Part of getting the sugar out of your diet means you have to treat breakfast as what it really is: the most important meal of the day. Breakfast literally means the break to the fast you experienced since last night's dinner or snack. That's why it's so important. What you have (or don't have) for breakfast can essentially make or break your whole day. Don't be afraid to eat a well-rounded meal in the morning. By doing so, you might just find yourself experiencing more energy than you remembered was possible and getting rid of daily munchies, cravings, and the 10:00 A.M. sugar blues.

The human body really is an amazing machine. Give it the nutrients it requires and it treats you well. Start it with the right fuel in the morning and it runs efficiently all day long.

The tips in this chapter are designed to help you do just that. They'll teach you how to have a better breakfast that's low in sugar and high in taste.

breads and spreads

97. **Pick out bread that has the lowest amount of sugars per serving.** Don't forget that yeast-raised bread has sugar in it almost by definition. Sugar is added to make yeast multiply and to cause bread to rise. (This phenomenon is a good illustration of why sugar exacerbates yeast problems in those who have candidiasis.)

98. **Besides just knowing about bread's sugar content,** all sugar-conscious consumers should avoid the bleached flour that most commercial yeasted breads contain. Flour bleaching forms alloxan, a compound that has been shown to

cause diabetes in animals by destroying the beta cells of the pancreas.

99. **Whole-grain bread is a taste treat all on its own.** Its texture, flavor, and chewiness beat the blandness of refined white bread hands down. It's so satisfying there's simply no need to top its taste with a sugary jam.

100. **Sourdough is not only a great change of pace** but also is a sugar-free way of indulging in bread. Sourdough bread is naturally leavened with fermenting agents that break down the flour's cellulose structure, neutralize phytic acid (which makes the food's minerals less available to our bodies), and release more nutrients into the dough. The result is a more nutritious bread that has no sugar. Look for whole-grain varieties such as those from French Meadow Bakery and Pacific Bakery, which are sold in natural food stores throughout the country.

101. **Naturally leavened raisin bread** is a great alternative to a Danish or Pop-Tart for those still weaning themselves from sugar-started mornings. For some, it can even serve as dessert. One client of mine told me she could satisfy her yen for cookies by indulging in a slice of toasted, lightly buttered Kamut Almond-Raisin Bread from Pacific Bakery.

102. **Sprouted bread is a healthful, sweet way to start your day.** The germination process used to make the bread naturally converts some of the grain's starches to

sugars and produces a bread that's so good it's worth a special visit to your local health food store to buy it. Good brands include Essene Bread from Lifestream Natural Foods and Manna Bread from Nature's Path.

103. Toast bread to bring out its sweetness. If you've got to have a touch of sweetness, this is a great way to do it. Toasting bread converts just enough of its starches to sugars for more sweetness for your taste buds.

104. A dab of creamy butter adds a sweet touch that satisfies many. True, the butter supplies fat, but remember that a little fat is balancing to the blood sugar and improves the ratio of insulin to glucagon, which helps the body access its stored fat for energy.

105. For your own cinnamon toast, sprinkle cinnamon on top of the melted butter. You'll be amazed that this topping has no sugar.

106. Yogurt cheese is a delightful spread for bread as well. To make it, simply line a colander with cheesecloth, place a drip bowl underneath, and put two cups of plain, low-fat yogurt on top of the cheesecloth. Put everything in the refrigerator, let the yogurt drain for several hours or overnight, and what remains is delicious cheese that is a great toast topper.

107. Try to get out of the habit of using jam or fruit spread as a toast topper. An all-fruit spread is a better choice than a sugar-sweetened jam, but only because it uses natural sweeteners instead of refined sugar. Most people are amazed to find out that popular fruit-spread brands such as Polaner All-Fruit and Smucker's Simply Fruit usually contain the *same amount of sugars* as regular sugar-sweetened preserves. That's 8 to 12 grams of sugars in every tablespoon. *Three Sweet Teeth.* ۩ ۩ ۩

108. Low-sugar preserves usually contain about half the amount of sugars as regular preserves, but they're made with nutrient-depleting refined sugar and artificial colors. It's far better for you to buy an all-fruit spread and dilute it with water for your own low-sugar jam.

109. Unsweetened apple butter is a better choice than jam when you want something sweet. It contains less sugars than preserves—usually 4 to 7 grams per tablespoon—but be sure to use only a tablespoon or less. *Two Sweet Teeth.* ۩ ۩

110. Another way to get that fruit-sweet flavor with less sugar is to try Kozlowski Farms brand fruit spreads. Also sweetened with just fruit, Kozlowski Farms spreads have the lowest amount of sugars on the market—1 gram per tablespoon of spread—and are a boon for anyone who is used to jam but is really serious about lowering sugar intake. Call 707-887-1587 if you have trouble locating these spreads at natural food stores in your area, or check out www. kozlowskifarms.com. *One Sweet Tooth.* ۩

111. Or make your own homemade jam. Just blend and
heat the fruit of your choice, add sweet spices if you want,
and use as you would any other jam. This is a great way to
use up any fruit you have around the house. The variety of
possibilities of different fruit spreads that you can make are
endless, but here is one example from my former adminis-
trative assistant, Amy Bondi. *Two Sweet Teeth.* 🦷 🦷

PEACH BUTTER 🦷 🦷

2 fresh medium-sized peaches

Peel peaches and slice them into pieces. Add peach pieces to a
food processor or blender and whip until smooth. Heat blended
peaches on medium-high heat in a saucepan until boiling.
Then turn heat to low and simmer, stirring occasionally, until
mixture thickens to desired apple-butter-like consistency.
Makes ¼ cup. 🦷 🦷

112. Or make a veggie butter. Sweet spreads don't always
have to be made with fruit, you know. They can be just as
tasty when made with sweet vegetables such as carrots. The
following recipe might sound a little strange, but it's a delicious and nutritious alternative to fruit jam. This one
comes from *The Good Breakfast Book* by Nikki and David
Goldbeck. *One Sweet Tooth.* 🦷

CARROT BUTTER 🦷

1 cup cooked carrots
2 tablespoons nut butter (see tip 113)
1 teaspoon honey
¼ teaspoon salt (omit if nut butter is salted)

Puree one cup cooked carrots in a food processor or mash with a fork. Beat until smooth with nut butter of your choice, honey, and salt. *Makes ¾ cup.* 🦷

113. **Explore the world of nut and seed butters,** including everything from almond butter to tahini (sesame seed butter). Peanut butter is always a nutrition-packed favorite, but other butters can offer variety and lend their own special creaminess to your usual morning toast. Be sure to buy an *unsweetened* nut butter, though. Jif and Skippy just won't do it. Look for such brands as Arrowhead Mills, Maranatha Natural Foods, and Roaster Fresh by Kettle Foods.

* ***Bonus Tip*** See if your local health food store offers grind-your-own nut butters. Their extra-fresh taste can't be beat.

114. **Melted low-fat cheese** is another way to top your toast—the protein and fat will balance your blood sugar.

breakfast goodies

115. **Muffins can be a source of high-quality, balanced nutrition,** but most commercial brands are the furthest thing from this ideal, being sources of empty-calorie sugars and not much more. Be especially careful of fat-free varieties, which often have more sugars than many cookies and cakes.

116. **Check out your local natural food supermarket,** where you may be able to find homemade, naturally sweetened, but low-sugar goodies that are baked locally.

117. **Or bake your own.** After all, muffins really are quick breads, usually taking not much more than thirty minutes to make from start to finish. If you're unsure of how to use natural sweeteners in your baking, pay special attention to the "Tips for Better Baking" section in chapter 7, check out some of the fine cookbooks listed in the bibliography, and of course make sure to use my cookbooks for great recipes.

118. **Use sweet vegetables and fruits**—such as winter squash, bananas, or apples—to add natural sweetness and moisture to the muffins you bake. The following recipe, from my book *Hot Times*, uses grated zucchini and carrots and finely chopped apples in this way. *One Sweet Tooth.* 🦷

SUNBURST MUFFINS 🦷

1 cup milled flaxseeds
½ cup ground walnuts
¾ cup vanilla Fat Flush Whey Protein
2 teaspoons aluminum-free baking powder
1 teaspoon baking soda
1½ teaspoons cinnamon
⅛ teaspoon ginger
¼ teaspoon salt
4 teaspoons macadamia nut oil
2 eggs
¼ cup honey
2 teaspoons vanilla extract
⅓ cup grated zucchini
⅓ cup grated carrot
¼ cup finely chopped Granny Smith apple
or other baking apple
⅔ cup ricotta cheese
½ cup chopped walnuts (optional)
2 tablespoons finely chopped raisins or
cranberries (optional)

Preheat oven to 350 degrees. Lightly coat 12 muffin cups with
cooking spray. In a small bowl, whisk together the flaxseed,
walnuts, whey protein, baking powder, baking soda, cinnamon,
ginger, and salt. Set aside.

In a large mixing bowl, mix together the macadamia nut oil,
eggs, honey, vanilla, zucchini, carrot, apple, and ricotta. Fold
the flaxseed mixture into the egg mixture. Fold in the chopped

walnuts, if using, and the raisins, if using. Divide the batter into the muffin cups. (Cups will be almost full.)

Bake 18 to 20 minutes or until a toothpick inserted into middle of a muffin comes out clean. Let cool; store in refrigerator. Serve with a drizzle of honey, if desired. These muffins freeze very well. *Makes 12 regular or 36 miniature muffins.* 🦷

119. **Begin easily converting your own favorite muffin recipes** to more nutritious versions by replacing sugar with Sucanat, date "sugar," or brown rice syrup powder, and by using whole-wheat pastry flour in place of all-purpose flour.

120. **Use high-protein ingredients** such as nut butters, nuts, seeds, eggs, or "supergrains" such as quinoa, amaranth, or teff to balance out the sugar content of muffins. In this recipe, adapted from a recipe shared with us by the Arrowhead Mills company, peanut butter adds creamy flavor, moisture, and power-packed nutrition that will keep you going for hours. *Two Sweet Teeth.* 🦷 🦷

PEANUT BUTTER MUFFINS 🦷🦷

2 cups whole-wheat pastry flour
1 tablespoon baking powder
½ teaspoon sea salt (optional)
¼ cup natural-style peanut butter

⅓ cup oil
¼ cup honey or molasses
1½ cups rice milk or almond milk

Stir flour, baking powder, and salt in a bowl. Mix peanut butter, oil, honey, and rice milk in a separate large bowl until smooth. Add dry mixture to liquid mixture and mix with minimal strokes. Do not beat. Fill 12 oiled muffin tins two-thirds full. Bake in preheated 350°F oven 25 minutes or until done. *Makes 12 muffins.* 🦷 🦷

121. **Giving up familiar sweet foods can be difficult,** but it's not always because it's hard to give up all the sugars in these foods. Sometimes it's just because we're creatures of habit, accustomed to foods we grew up with or are used to. Instead of totally abstaining from traditional favorites, try this recipe from my book *Hot Times: How to Eat Well, Live Healthy, and Feel Sexy During the Change.* One Sweet Tooth. 🦷

BANANA FRENCH TOAST 🦷

2 eggs
2 large ripe bananas
1 scoop vanilla Fat Flush Whey Protein
½ cup water
½ teaspoon cinnamon
1 teaspoon vanilla extract
6 slices wheat-free, yeast-free spelt bread
(French Meadow HealthSeed Spelt)

Blend the eggs, bananas, whey protein, water, cinnamon, and vanilla in a blender or food processor until smooth. Pour the mixture into a 9-by-13-inch pan. Place the bread in the banana mixture and let soak until the liquid is mostly absorbed, about 15 minutes, turning the bread occasionally.

Lightly coat a large heavy skillet with olive oil spray; heat over medium heat. Add the bread and cook until golden brown, about 3 to 4 minutes per side. Freezes well. *Serves 6.* 🦷

pancake paradise

122. Don't give up pancakes just because you have to give up white flour and white sugar. Try whole-grain varieties instead and you'll never again want to go back to those made with all-purpose flour. Two convenience products that can help you enjoy with little fuss the delightful, light, almost nutty flavor of whole-grain pancakes are Arrowhead Mills' Multi-Grain Pancake Mix and Bob's Red Mill 10-Grain Mix.

123. Take any basic pancake recipe and put your own stamp on it. By using different herbs, spices, fruit, flavoring extracts, and unrefined oils, you can make the pancakes different every time you make them, depending upon your mood, and you'll be adding flavor without refined sugar. The only thing stopping your culinary creations is the inhibition of your imagination.

124. **Add ¼ teaspoon pumpkin pie spice** to the pancakes and have your own Thanksgiving.

125. **Make the cakes maple-y.** Include some natural maple flavoring and a teaspoon or two of maple syrup for a whole new flavor. *One Sweet Tooth.* 🦷

126. **Add some fresh blueberries to the pancake batter.** Practically no one can resist fresh blueberry pancakes right off the griddle. *One Sweet Tooth.* 🦷

127. **Simply add a few drops of vanilla** for a sweeter taste.

128. **Go nutty.** If you're nuts about almonds, use expeller-pressed almond oil in the recipe and a dash of almond extract. Top with almond butter or home-toasted sliced almonds for pure almond joy. Get the idea? Now let your creativity guide you.

129. **Baby food isn't just for babies.** It also happens to be a special secret ingredient in many successful sugar-free sensations. (Shh! Don't tell anyone. Word might get around.) If you're on the run and don't have time to spend all morning in the kitchen, try "babying" yourself with the luxury of these little helpers, as Melissa Diane Smith, nutritionist and author of *Going Against the Grain,* has done in this recipe. Brown rice flour is used here to allow the special sweetness of the sweet potato to shine through. *One Sweet Tooth.* 🦷

MELISSA'S SWEET POTATO PANCAKES 🦷

1 egg (or 1½ teaspoons Ener-G Egg Replacer
mixed in 2 tablespoons water)
1 4-ounce jar Earth's Best sweet potato baby food
1½ tablespoons expeller-pressed oil
¼ cup water
¾ cup brown rice flour

Preheat a nonstick skillet over medium heat. Beat the egg lightly and add baby food and oil. Add the water to the emptied baby food jar, cover, shake it a couple of times, and empty its contents into the liquid ingredients to get all of the baby food out of the jar; then mix well. Add the brown rice flour and mix again. Drop batter into 2-inch-round pancakes and cook until brown on one side. Flip over, push the pancakes down, and cook until done. *Serves 2 to 3.* 🦷

Variation: If you want the pancakes to taste more nutty instead of creamy, add ¼ cup finely chopped pecans to the batter right before cooking.

130. **Say good-bye to Aunt Jemima pancake syrup (and others like it).** The first three ingredients in the original syrup are corn syrup, sugar syrup, and high-fructose corn syrup—all refined sweeteners that are nutrient-depleted as well as nutrient-depleting.

131. **Reach for 100** percent pure maple syrup if you must top your pancakes with something sweet. Sure, maple syrup is high in natural sugars, but it also contains nutrients that

the imitation syrups just don't have. In addition, it has a distinctive, robust taste that can't be beat. Maple syrup is very concentrated, though—1 tablespoon contains 13 grams of sugars—so get into the habit of dabbing it on pancakes one drop at a time.

132. Or use maple syrup diluted with water or almond milk. Pure maple syrup is so concentrated that most people will want less on their pancakes if they taste their food before they pour the syrup on. But if you always pour on more than you need, dilute the syrup first.

133. Unsweetened applesauce also tops pancakes well, but try not to use more than ½ cup (which is one fruit exchange) on your stack of cakes. For a sweet change of pace, explore the different varieties of unsweetened fruit applesauces, such as strawberry applesauce or peach applesauce from Solana Gold or Santa Cruz Natural.

134. Try to use fruit instead of syrups and spreads on pancakes. Whether chopped, sliced, whole, or blended, fruit is nature's most perfect sweetener.

---

breakfast entrées

135. Have a substantial breakfast that includes adequate protein and fiber if you have blood sugar problems. If high-sugar foods make up your meal, you're apt to spend the rest of the day with erratic blood sugar levels, not feeling well and prone to going into munchie mayhem.

136. Enjoy some eggs-ceptional breakfasts. Eggs are a nearly perfect food that has gotten an unfair rap from the media and some health professionals recently. While eggs do contain cholesterol, dietary cholesterol only becomes a problem when it becomes altered because of smoking, curing, or aging processes, as in such foods as sausage, aged cheese, and meats. Enjoy eggs in moderation and use them as great sources of protein to balance blood sugar quickly.

137. Another reason to eat eggs is that they may very well help blood sugar metabolism. You see, each insulin molecule that works to balance blood sugar contains eight atoms of sulfur, a trace mineral that eggs supply in abundance. Many antidiabetic drugs also contain sulfur, so it's reasonable to assume that eating sulfur-rich foods such as eggs can help your insulin work more effectively.

138. Tired of eggs and toast? For an exotic twist to your usual morning meal, try it the Oriental way. Fry up leftover brown rice and a scrambled egg in two teaspoons of rice bran or sesame oil. Top with green onion tops and a bit of parsley if you like or a dash of dark sesame oil. This dish gives you complex carbohydrates, protein, and healthy fat—everything you need to begin your day the balanced blood sugar way!

139. **Skip the ham or bacon.** Although they contain protein, they also contain entirely too much sugar as well as saturated fat, altered (or oxidized) cholesterol, and potentially carcinogenic chemicals.

140. **To replace high-sugar sausage** (which is also high in fat and salt), make your own. Use lean ground turkey or ground beef and add flavorful herbs such as garlic and fennel. Here's an example shared with me by author and nutritionist Melissa Diane Smith:

HOMEMADE TURKEY SAUSAGE

1 pound lean ground turkey (Shelton's brand preferred)
2–6 garlic cloves, pressed
½ teaspoon rubbed sage
½ teaspoon ground fennel

Preheat oven to 350 degrees. Mix the above ingredients, shape the meat mixture into 2-inch-round sausage patties, and place on a broiler pan or on a wire rack above a baking pan. Bake until done and no pink remains in the center, about 20–25 minutes. Add sea salt to taste at the table if necessary. *Serves 3 to 4.*

141. **Expand your breakfast repertoire.** Break through the bonds of traditional breakfast foods. Your morning meal doesn't have to consist of eggs, sausage, toast, or cereal. It can be anything that's low in sugar and that gets you off to

a good start. Leftovers from last night's dinner work well in a pinch.

142. **Cooked chicken, turkey, or lean beef can fill your protein bill** when you have no eggs left in the fridge.

143. **Or try low-fat cottage cheese.** If you don't like it plain, try adding cinnamon on top for a sweeter taste.

cereals and milks to top them

144. **Cereals are one of the top places you need to watch out for sugars.** Hidden in some of the healthiest-looking cereals are sugars in every disguised form imaginable. Review the list of sugar names in tip 79 before you shop for cereals and be sure to pick out a whole-grain brand with 3 grams of sugars or less per serving if at all possible.

145. **Stick with basics** such as unsweetened shredded wheat and unsweetened oatmeal. They may not be fancy but they offer wholesome, sugar-free nutrition.

146. **Cream of wheat and cream of rice** are also good choices, but make sure to buy the whole-grain varieties (such as Arrowhead Mills' Bear Mush and Rice 'n Shine, Bob's Red Mill Creamy Wheat and Creamy Rice Cereals, or Lundberg Farms Rice Cereal). Popular commercial brands of these cereals that are made from refined grains

lack fiber and many nutrients found in the original grain and raise the blood sugar quickly.

147. **If you grab sugar-rich, ready-to-eat cereals** because you simply don't have time to make hot whole-grain cereals in the morning, then make them the night before—in the oven, that is! There's nothing nicer than waking up to the smell of cooked whole-grain cereal that's ready for you to eat. Here is an overnight recipe for cooking cereal grains that I learned from my 106-year-old mentor, Dr. Hazel Parcells.

OVERNIGHT WHOLE-GRAIN CEREAL 🦷

2½ cups boiling water
1 cup grains (rolled oats, cornmeal, cracked wheat,
barley grits, or brown rice)
1 teaspoon salt

In a casserole, pour the boiling water over the grains and add the salt. Preheat oven to 350 degrees. Place casserole in oven and reduce heat to 200 degrees. The cereal will cook in about two hours, or it may remain in the oven all day or all night at 200 degrees without reducing the nutritional value. To make larger quantities, use the same proportions of liquids to dry materials. *Serves 4.* 🦷

148. **Use natural liquid sweeteners sparingly,** by the drop, on your cereals. A little molasses, honey, or maple syrup can go a long, long way.

149. Better yet, use fruit as a natural cereal sweetener. A few sliced peaches, strawberries, or blueberries can brighten your bowl.

150. Granola may seem like a health food, but its sugar content often puts it in the same league as many desserts. Be careful which brand you buy, or make your own so you can control its sugar content. Try the following recipe, which is one of my favorites in *The Yeast Connection Cookbook* by William Crook, M.D., and Marjorie Hurt Jones, R.N. It is the lowest-sugar granola I have ever seen, but it is still absolutely delicious. *One Sweet Tooth.* 🦷

OAT GRANOLA 🦷

3 cups rolled oats
½ cup sunflower seeds
½ cup almonds, halved or coarsely chopped
1–2 teaspoons ground cinnamon
¼ teaspoon salt (optional)
¼ cup oil
¼ cup pineapple juice
½ cup mashed banana

Preheat oven to 350 degrees. Combine oats, seeds, almonds, cinnamon, and salt in a large mixing bowl. In a blender jar, combine the oil, pineapple juice, and mashed banana and blend briefly. Pour the thick liquid over the oat mixture and blend well. Spread

on a large jelly-roll pan and bake for about 40–45 minutes, stirring the granola two or three times. When lightly brown, remove
from the oven—it crisps as it cools. Store the cooled granola in
tightly capped glass jars, in a cool place. *Makes about 6 cups.* 🦷

151. **Toss together your own muesli** and eliminate altogether the honey, maple syrup, and fruit juice used to
sweeten granola. Muesli really is a hodgepodge, and it can
be as individualistic as you are. Common muesli ingredients to include in any way you see fit are uncooked rolled
oats, corn or wheat flakes, unsweetened puffed cereals such
as puffed rice, seeds and chopped nuts, and chopped fruit
such as apples or dried fruit such as raisins or dates.

152. **Milk may seem like a natural,** but remember it's naturally high in milk sugars. In 1 cup of milk there's 11 grams
of sugars, so go easy using it on your cereal.

153. **Lactose-reduced milk** can help eliminate the unwanted
bloating and digestive upset milk can cause in most of the
world's population. Unfortunately, though, the sugars in
this product are even more rapidly absorbed than the sugars naturally present in milk and can cause blood sugar
problems. Diabetics especially need to beware.

154. **Almond milk, soy milk, and rice milk** are helpful for
people who have trouble digesting cow's milk, and they can
substitute for milk as cereal toppers and recipe ingredients.
But keep in mind that they mostly consist of sugars, just

like milk. Using any type of sugar-rich milk on a sweet cereal can send your blood sugar soaring (and then falling), so use all milks judiciously. You can make sugar-free almond milk at home by following the recipe below from my book *Hot Times. Two Sweet Teeth.* 🦷 🦷

ALMOND MILK 🦷 🦷

1 cup boiling water
½ cup ground almonds or almond meal (or a commercial product called Ener-G Nut-Quik)

Pour the water over the ground almonds and let steep for 10 minutes; blend. Pour through a sieve that has been placed over a small bowl. *Makes about ¾ cup.* 🦷 🦷

breakfast beverages

155. The best drink to begin your day is pure, filtered water. It's the perfect sugar-free antidote for your thirst and for your body, which has been without it all night long.

156. Just say no to juice as a breakfast beverage. Although it may seem like the ultimate in a healthy drink, whether it's from a container or straight from your juicer, juice is one of the quickest ways to give your pancreas a shock and throw your blood sugar so off-kilter that you might feel out of balance all day long. In one 8-ounce glass of apple juice, for example, you get all of the natural sugars from the 3½ pounds of apples used to make the juice and none of the blood-sugar-balancing fiber. If your start your morning this way, you may experience an initial high, but you're sure to suffer from an eventual blood sugar low that will leave you wanting more sugar.

157. **If you can't give up juice just yet,** gradually begin diluting fruit or vegetable juice with more and more water to wean yourself away from the high-sugar content of straight juice. In time, you'll find that a little juice goes very far.

158. **Use herbal tea** as another, more interesting way to thin out juice. One client of mine begins her day with iced Red Zinger and a little bit of pomegranate juice, while another goes for mint tea with a touch of apple juice. The choices really are endless. Be creative and see what tasty drink concoctions you can devise to lessen your juice intake.

159. **If you think you're doing well to gulp down an instant breakfast drink in the morning,** think again. No matter how many nutrients a drink mix such as Carnation Instant Breakfast may contain, it doesn't do you much good when there are twenty-two grams of sugars per serving. It's better for you to make a smoothie that is fruity and unbelievably delicious such as this one from my *Eat Fat Lose Weight* book and swallow a good, sugar-free multivitamin. *Three Sweet Teeth.* 🦷 🦷 🦷

BERRY NUT SMOOTHIE 🦷🦷🦷

1 cup frozen blueberries
¼ cup frozen strawberries
1¾ cups water
4 tablespoons nonfat plain yogurt
2 tablespoons flax oil
2 tablespoons almond butter
2 scoops whey protein powder
1 cup ice

Place ingredients in a blender. Blend until creamy, approximately 2 to 3 minutes. *Makes four 8-ounce servings.* 🦷🦷🦷

160. **If you're looking for one more reason to convince yourself to give up coffee,** this may be it: Coffee is bad for your blood sugar. It provides a temporary lift but taxes your pancreas and adrenals, which control your blood-sugar-balancing mechanisms. It also causes blood-sugar-balancing minerals to be washed out of your system. Chalk up these reasons and you might just have enough incentive to give up coffee for good.

161. **Coffee with sugar is double trouble.** Not only does the sugar stimulate the pancreas into activity, but the caffeine prompts the adrenals to induce the liver to convert its stored energy into even more sugar in the bloodstream. Essentially, it's a sugar double whammy! If you feel you must drink coffee, give your pancreas a break: Cut down on the amount you drink, switch to the water-

> * **Bonus Tip** Coffee substitutes made out of such ingredients as chicory and dandelion roots are tasty ways to help satisfy the desire for a coffee-like taste without the caffeine of coffee.

process decaffeinated variety, and learn to drink it without sweetening.

162. **Flavored coffees are quite the rage these days,** but guess what most of them are flavored with? Sugar, of course—that nasty five-letter word. In place of sugar, try adding natural flavoring extracts to decaf coffee and coffee substitutes to give them that gourmet flair. Here's one tasty example.

FRENCH VANILLA CAFÉ 🦷

Boiling water
1 roasted dandelion root or chicory tea bag
½ teaspoon vanilla extract

Pour boiling water over the tea bag in a coffee cup and let it steep for 5–10 minutes. Add vanilla and stir. *Serves 1.* 🦷

get the sugar out of soups and salads

S oups and salads are versatile foods. They can be eaten by themselves for a snack or light lunch, together for a more substantial meal, or as starters before a main course. They can also be made to satisfy our desire for all kinds of tastes and textures. Soups, for example, can be comforting and creamy, clear and spicy, or stewlike and chunky. Salads can vary from crisp and crunchy (as in the case of a lettuce- and vegetable-based salad) to chewy (as in the case of a grain-based salad).

With so much room for variation, it's understandable how soups and salads can become either sources of lots of hidden sugar or foods that are practically sugar-free. The difference depends on what kinds of ingredients go into your soup pot or salad bowl. Is the soup made from homemade stock or from sugar-containing commercial stock? Are a variety of fresh vegetables and herbs added to flavor the soup, or such ingredients as dextrose and high-fructose corn syrup? Is the dressing on your fresh salad a homemade vinaigrette or a store-bought honey Dijon?

Start to ask questions like these about the soups and salads you consume and utilize the tips in this chapter. Low-sugar soup-and-salad eating suddenly will become a lot easier.

Soups and salads should showcase all the goodness fresh vegetables (and sometimes meat and grains) can offer. Use high-quality ingredients and get the sugar out of them. Not only will soups and salads become more enjoyable, but they will also be healthful.

soup basics

163. **It never ceases to amaze me how manufacturers sneak sugar into our most basic food staples.** Take chicken stock, for example. This is a versatile ingredient for a health-oriented kitchen, but if you look over the top brands in commercial supermarket aisles, it's difficult to find one that doesn't include some type of sugar. (Sugar in soups usually comes disguised as dextrose, maltodextrin, corn syrup solids, or high-fructose corn syrup.) To avoid the hidden sugar, make your own poultry stock in a Crock-Pot or on top of the stove and taste the superior flavor of homemade stock as it was meant to be—without any sugar. Here's a handed-down recipe some of my staff use.

BASIC CHICKEN OR TURKEY STOCK

2–4 pounds chicken or turkey parts
(wings, backs, necks, and giblets work well)
1 bay leaf (optional)
1 celery stalk with leaves, chopped (optional)
1 large onion, quartered (optional)

Put all the ingredients in a large pot with a lid and cover with cold water. Bring slowly to a boil. Once it boils, reduce the heat, cover, and simmer for 1½ to 3 hours. (Longer cooking produces a more flavorful stock.) Cool stock to room temperature. Remove the poultry parts and vegetables and strain the stock. Refrigerate overnight or until the fat has solidified on top. Remove the fat and store the stock in the freezer in the size containers you use most frequently. *Makes about 8 cups.*

164. **If convenience is important to you,** seek out sugarless canned chicken broth available from the Shelton's, Hain, and Health Valley companies.

165. **Don't throw away the water over which you've steamed vegetables.** Save it for use as a light, inexpensive, sugar-free vegetable broth to add to soups and stir-fries.

166. **Or use an instant vegetable broth mix** such as those from Bernard Jensen, or Dr. Bronner's, which are available in most health food stores. Also try Rapunzel Pure Organics

(www.rapunzel.com) and Edward and Sons Trading Co. (www.edwardandsons.com).

167. **Add chopped vegetables of your choice to any sugar-free stock** to create an ultraquick vegetable soup. Just bring the broth to a boil, add the vegetables, and simmer, covered, for twenty to thirty minutes.

168. **Or try Tabatchnick vegetable-based soups,** which are available in the frozen foods section of many grocery stores. They contain so many wholesome ingredients that their taste is close to the flavor of homemade soup, and they have no added sugar.

169. **Use whole-grain noodles or brown rice** when making chicken noodle or rice soup. The extra minerals supplied by these whole-grain products are a bonus for your blood sugar control systems.

170. **Or buy Hain sugar-free soups** to have on hand.

171. **Be cautious when buying fat-free soups.** Remember, fat-free doesn't necessarily mean sugar-free. Instead, it often means that ingredients such as sugar, corn syrup, honey, and fruit juice have replaced the fat.

172. **Whole-wheat, oat, brown rice, or chickpea flour** can thicken a cream soup just as nicely as all-purpose flour—and more nutritiously.

173. **Sweet starchy vegetables such as squash can thicken cream soup** or even make a creamlike soup all by themselves. Here's a simple, slightly sweet, and utterly creamy recipe I came up with for my book *Hot Times. One Sweet Tooth.* 🦷

BUTTERNUT BISQUE 🦷

4 cups water

1 large butternut squash, peeled and cubed

¼ teaspoon salt (optional)

¼ teaspoon cumin

¼ teaspoon coriander

¼ teaspoon grated ginger

¼ teaspoon garlic powder

6 parsley sprigs

12 toasted almonds

6 heaping tablespoons nonfat plain yogurt

Place the water and squash in a soup pot. Cover and simmer for 5 minutes. Add the salt, if using, cumin, coriander, ginger, and garlic powder. Continue simmering for 15 minutes. Puree in a blender or food processor. Serve garnished with parsley sprigs, almonds, and dollops of yogurt. *Serves 6.* 🦷

salad days

174. Salads are naturally low in sugar and good for your blood sugar. When they're chock-full of dark green leafy lettuce and vegetables ranging from artichoke hearts to zucchini, salads are loaded with vitamins and minerals that your body needs to maintain optimal blood sugar levels.

> **✳ *Bonus Tip*** Judge the nutrition of your salad by the richness of its color. Pale iceberg lettuce is much lower in minerals than its darker green cousins and, therefore, not as helpful for your blood sugar. If you're used to iceberg lettuce, try adding a few darker green lettuce leaves (such as red or green leaf or romaine) to your regular salad to increase its nutritional content.

175. Buy the freshest ingredients possible so your salad is flavorful all on its own. When your vegetables are crunchy and tasty, you'll want to taste more of them and less of a sugar-containing dressing.

176. Add some interest to your salad by including some vegetables you haven't tried before. Any vegetable you would add to salad is essentially sugar-free, so feel free to experiment.

177. **If you're looking for some sweetness in your bowl of greens,** try using grated carrots or beets. Both are amazingly sweet and add vibrant color to your salad as well. *One Sweet Tooth.* 🦷

178. **As an herb or as a vegetable,** fennel brings its subtly sweet, licorice-like flavor to any food it accompanies. For a change of pace in your salad, try adding sliced strips of fresh fennel.

179. **Have you ever tried jicama?** If not, you're missing a real treat. Naturally sweet, crisp, and mild, jicama is a tuber-like vegetable that is eaten raw and is a special addition to salads for many people. Try it the next time you get an opportunity.

180. **Croutons and bacon bits are the only weak links** in the otherwise sugar-free typical salad fare. Hiding in these salad toppers are sugar and high-fructose corn syrup. If you really want croutons, make them at home by adding herbs and garlic to whole-grain bread cubes and oven-toasting them, but skip the bacon bits altogether.

181. **Adding leftover strips of chicken or turkey or flaked tuna** to a salad can make a satisfying, sugar-free meal-in-one that's especially nice for lunch on a hot summer day.

182. **Pasta salad is a light meal—light on nutrition, that is.** Believe it or not, the refined pasta found in most commercial salads is, nutritionally, almost in the same category as sugar: It supplies calories but few nutrients. To increase

the mineral and fiber content of this meal and to help your blood sugar, be sure to use whole-grain pasta.

183. **You can also take your favorite pasta salad recipe** and use leftover whole grains in place of the pasta. Brown rice, bulgur, barley, and quinoa all work well in pasta-salad recipes.

dressed for success

184. **A salad dressing is one place sugar grams can pile up quickly** if you don't choose with care the dressing you use. Watch out for hidden sugars in all dressings, but especially try to avoid fat-free ones made with fruit juices or honey.

185. **If you're used to honey-based dressings,** wean yourself away from commercial brands that have additional sugars in them and start yourself off with a naturally sweet homemade dressing such as this wondrous tasty twist you've just gotta try from my *Eat Fat Lose Weight Cookbook. Two Sweet Teeth.* 🦷 🦷

ORANGE-SESAME DRESSING 🦷 🦷

¼ cup fresh orange juice
2 tablespoons apple cider vinegar
¼ cup extra-virgin olive oil

1 teaspoon sesame oil
Salt and pepper
6 teaspoons sesame seeds, for topping

Whisk orange juice, vinegar, and oils together. Season with salt and pepper to taste. Drizzle over salad, and sprinkle each serving of salad with approximately 1 teaspoon of sesame seeds. *Makes ½ cup.* 🦷 🦷

186. **Gradually thin out sweet dressings,** such as the one above, with water as your taste and desire for sweets lessen. *One Sweet Tooth.* 🦷

187. **Vinegar and oil are a tried-and-true dressing.** Simple and delicious, a dressing of just oil and vinegar is one of the best ways to stay away from hidden sugars in your dressing.

> ✳ ***Bonus Tip*** There are a lot of vinegars from which to choose, and each one gives its own unique flavor. Some nice ones to try are balsamic vinegar, red wine vinegar, and rice vinegar.

188. **Make an herb vinegar** for an extra-special dressing ingredient. To make it, fill a glass bottle or jar with approximately 1 cup of fresh herbs such as dill, thyme, rosemary, or tarragon. Add 1 quart of cider vinegar, red wine vinegar, or white vinegar, cap the bottle and label it, and let it stand in a cool, dark place. After three to four weeks, it's ready to use.

189. **Avoid fruit-flavored vinegars such as raspberry or blueberry vinegar.** Both fruit and refined sugar are used to flavor these trendy salad toppers.

190. **The sweetness and sourness of lemon or lime juices** are naturals in salad dressings. Combine them with olive oil and crushed garlic or herbs if you wish to make a healthy dressing to season your salad.

191. **If you want a bit more pizzazz added to lemon and oil,** try using sugar-free mustard as I did in this classic easy-to-make dressing from my first book, *Beyond Pritikin*.

FRENCH OLIVE OIL DRESSING

½ cup extra-virgin olive oil
2 tablespoons fresh lemon juice
1 teaspoon Dijon mustard
¼ teaspoon salt (optional)

Put all the ingredients in a small covered jar. Shake vigorously for 30 seconds and refrigerate. Remove from the refrigerator at least an hour before serving to liquefy the oil. *Makes ½ cup.*

192. **Transform your oil into a salad dressing all by itself** through the art of herbal infusion. Follow tip 47. Olive oil makes a particularly good herbed oil.

193. **Or transform your oil by vigorously shaking it with tasty herbs.** Here's an example: In a small, covered jar,

put ½ cup sesame or peanut oil, 1½ tablespoons finely chopped ginger, 1 tablespoon chopped parsley, and 1 minced . clove of garlic. Shake the ingredients well and pour on top of your salad.

194. **Salsa by itself or combined with canola oil makes a quick, terrific dressing** that gives a definite kick to your salad greens.

195. **A nice change of pace is an avocado-based dressing.** I think you'll like this tried-and-true one. *One Sweet Tooth.* 🦷

GARLICKY AVOCADO DRESSING 🦷

2 small avocados, peeled, pitted, and mashed
2 teaspoons garlic, minced
4 tablespoons fresh lemon juice
4 tablespoons flaxseed oil

Mix all ingredients together in a bowl until well combined. Use immediately or store in fridge for up to 4 days. *Makes ½ cup.* 🦷

196. **Greek Tzatziki Sauce,** a cooling sauce that combines cucumber, herbs, and unsweetened yogurt, can make a refreshingly different salad dressing either by itself or mixed with water, oil, or lemon juice. It's simple to prepare, too.

GREEK TZATZIKI SAUCE 🦷

⅓ cucumber, peeled, seeded, and diced
1 cup plain low-fat yogurt
1 clove garlic, minced, *or* 1 green onion, chopped
1 tablespoon fresh dill weed *or* 1½ teaspoons dried dill weed *or*
1 tablespoon fresh mint *or* 1½ teaspoons dried mint

Combine all the ingredients in a bowl, cover, and chill for a few hours. *Makes 1 cup.* 🦷

197. If you're used to making a dressing from a mix, did you know that sugar is a component of almost all of those handy mixes? One exception is the Spice Hunter, which makes a complete line of mixes that are both salt- and sugar-free.

198. Two good bottled salad dressing lines to try are Cardini's and Paula's, both of which are found in natural food stores. Both lines contain no sugar and have several delicious varieties from which to choose. (Don't choose Paula's No-Oil Dressings, though. Like many fat-free dressings, these *do* contain sugar.)

get the sugar out of entrées and side dishes

*g*etting the sugar out of entrées and side dishes involves a shift in thinking. Instead of worrying about every drop of even naturally occurring fat in the foods you serve, your focus should turn to eliminating processed convenience foods that contain refined carbohydrates and hidden sugars. Doing so will not only help get the sugar out of your diet but also help get the fats you should avoid out of your diet as well. (Packaged foods that contain hidden sugars often contain harmful trans fats such as hydrogenated oils as well.)

If you stop to think about it, our ancestors survived very nicely eating whatever animal products and plant foods they could find. What they didn't eat was a continual supply of hidden sugar—and this is where Americans have gotten into trouble.

No one wants to spend all day cooking in the kitchen, but when TV dinners and mixes such as Hamburger Helper make up your meals, sugar becomes one of the biggest components of your diet. So what are you to do?

If, like most people, you value convenience above all else, the answer is to find smart ways of enjoying convenience without all that sugar. One way to do that is to plan ahead and make your own convenience foods. Roasting a turkey breast on Sunday afternoon doesn't take a lot of effort, but it can give you ready-to-use, sugar-free turkey meat that will be a godsend later on in the week for making quick sandwiches and such dishes as turkey tetrazzini or turkey hash. Making extra portions of such dishes as lasagna and stir-fries doesn't take much more work, but it can give you a way to enjoy heat-and-serve complete meals when you come home from work and are just too tired to cook.

Another way of coping is to seek out brands of products that give you equal convenience but far superior nutrition than the commercial brands. Finding these products sometimes means making a visit to your local natural food store, but the rewards you receive (less sugar, more nutrition, better taste, and convenience) make it well worth the trip.

Unlike other diet plans that you might have followed, getting the sugar out of the entrées and side dishes you eat does not in the slightest involve deprivation. In fact, it means experiencing more pure pleasure by eating delicious, fresher-tasting lunches and dinners than before. You can eat "real food" again—food that is wholesome, satisfying, and truly energizing. And you can enjoy a variety of dinners, from a broiled steak, baked potato, and salad to a chicken-and-vegetable stir-fry to black beans and brown rice.

Getting the sugar out of entrées and side dishes is not that difficult or mysterious, really. The more you stick with unprocessed natural foods (such as the ones recommended in this chapter), the less of a problem sugar will be.

meaty matters

199. **Meat has received so much bad press in the last decade** that many people are afraid to eat even small amounts. That's unfortunate because, as I explain in my book *Your Body Knows Best*, some people just can't thrive without it. Sure, meat contains some naturally occurring fat, but our bodies are designed to deal with some fat. It's sugar that's the real troublemaker.

200. **Stick with unprocessed meat** that is baked, broiled, sautéed, or stir-fried. Meat starts to cause problems with your health when it is highly processed—fried, smoked, cured, or aged and loaded with salt and sugar. Avoid meat products with concealed sugar—hot dogs, sausage, ham, and luncheon meats such as bologna and pastrami.

201. **Go ahead and have a lean cut of steak.** It's the steak sauce you should be more concerned about. Some steak sauces have up to 8 grams of sugars per tablespoon. If you use 2 tablespoons, that's the sugar equivalent of putting ½ cup of chocolate pudding on your steak!

202. **Eating lean red meat and poultry** is one of the best ways to perk up malfunctioning adrenal glands, an increas-

* **Bonus Tip** The antibiotics and hormones used to produce most meat these days pose potential problems for your health. Whenever possible, buy organically raised meats that are free of these harmful chemicals. Some poultry brands that offer organically raised chickens and turkeys are Shelton Farms, Harmony Farms, Foster Farms, and Young's Farm. Brands of beef to look for include Coleman Natural Meats and Ranch Foods Direct. Ranch Foods Direct is a specialty meat company selling natural beef—raised without hormones or antibiotics—along with natural poultry, buffalo, eggs, cheese, pork, lamb, seafood, and many other high-quality food items. Rancher Mike Callicrate opened the Colorado Springs business in 2003 to combine the best of traditional animal husbandry practices with an innovative processing method that rinses the blood from the meat during processing. Readers of this book can receive a special offer: a 10 percent discount on all of Mike's products. Please visit his Web site, www.ranchfoodsdirect.com, and then call 1-866-866-6328 to place your order. Mike's staff can send you a more complete listing with more elaborate offerings. To qualify for the special discount, please use the code ALG.

ingly common problem among people who are overstressed and overworked. This is important because the adrenal glands are intimately involved in sugar metabolism. By eating such foods as lean meats, which help your adrenals function better, you help stabilize your blood sugar levels.

203. Beef, pork, lamb, chicken, and turkey are all significant sources of zinc, a mineral that is crucial to proper blood sugar functioning but one that is deficient in more than 60 percent of the American population. (Beef and lamb, the meats people have been avoiding the most recently, are the two highest sources.) Not only is zinc an essential mineral for optimal adrenal function, but it also helps the beta cells of the pancreas store and release insulin as required. Pancreatic tissues of diabetics have been shown to have one-third the zinc of those of nondiabetics. Do your pancreas a favor and don't hesitate to eat small but frequent portions of these zinc-rich, sugar-free foods.

> ✳ *Bonus Tip* Whether you eat more lean poultry or heavier red meats should depend a lot on your metabolism. My book *Your Body Knows Best* goes into this in great detail, but generally, individuals who have slow metabolisms feel much better eating such lean animal products as white-meat chicken and turkey, while people with fast metabolisms tend to thrive on higher-fat lamb and beef.

204. If the idea of eating meat is hard for you to swallow, consider this: Eating meat causes your body to release glucagon, the hormone that works in direct opposition to insulin and helps your body burn off fat stores. Eating fare such as pasta, potatoes, and bread causes the pancreas to release more insulin, which can lead to erratic blood sugar highs and lows and, in many people, can really add on the pounds. While too much meat in the diet can be bad for your health, too little meat can be just as harmful. Two 3-ounce portions per day is a good amount for most people. (As an easy guide, a 3-ounce portion is the size of a deck of cards.)

205. Don't skip eating meat to make room for dessert. Although this plan sounds as if it would work calorie-wise, it's likely to backfire on you. You see, eating lean meat is one of the best ways to meet your daily protein requirements. Without adequate protein to help stabilize your blood sugar and energy levels, your body will crave and you will probably overeat high-carbohydrate foods such as sugar-rich desserts to give you the quick energy you are lacking.

206. Combine just a small amount of lean meat (3 ounces or so) with lots of vegetables (as you do in stir-fries and fajitas) to create a naturally balanced meal that's both low in sugars and stabilizing for your blood sugar.

207. Tacos can be a low-sugar, balanced meal as long as you avoid commercial taco-seasoning mixes that contain sugar. One brand that doesn't contain sugar is Hain Taco Seasoning Mix. Or instead of a mix you can use 1 teaspoon chili powder and ½ teaspoon onion powder to season 1 pound ground meat.

208. If you shake and then bake your chicken, you might be surprised to learn that bleached flour and four types of sugars are listed in the original Shake 'n Bake recipe mix. You will be pleasantly surprised with the Fat Flush version of fried chicken—the herbs lend flavor and health value. Tarragon is a good source of potassium, while rosemary pro-vides adds antioxidant power. Parsley is mineral-rich, and garlic will fight off the vampires. Here's a way to coat and bake your chicken without all that sugar. *One Sweet Tooth.* 🦷

CRISPY UNFRIED CHICKEN 🦷

¾ cup no-salt-added chicken broth
1 tablespoon olive oil
1 cup toasted wheat germ
1 teaspoon dried tarragon
1 teaspoon dried rosemary, crushed
1 teaspoon fresh parsley, chopped
1 teaspoon garlic powder
Salt to taste
4 (5-ounce) chicken thighs, skinned

Preheat oven to 350 degrees. In a small bowl, place the chicken broth and olive oil. In another bowl mix together the wheat germ, tarragon, rosemary, parsley, garlic powder, and salt. Dip the thighs, one at a time, in the broth-oil mixture, then coat with the wheat germ mixture. Bake until brown and cooked through, about 45–55 minutes. *Serves 4.* 🦷

209. Ever wonder what's in those TV dinners you heat up in the oven? Hidden sugars galore, unfortunately (not to mention hydrogenated oils and questionable preservatives), even in the "healthy" brands. The only meat-containing frozen dinners I can recommend are Shelton's whole-wheat chicken or turkey potpies, both of which are sugar-free.

go fish

210. Fried fish is a no-no for many reasons, not the least of which is that the batter that coats the fish usually contains white flour and white sugar. Better to go for baked, broiled, or poached fish instead.

211. Or make your own batter and oven-"fry" fish. Dipping fish in an egg wash or oil and then coating it with whole-grain flour, ground-up nuts or seeds, and a variety of herbs makes for a much tastier breading, and you won't even miss the hidden sugar normally found in this entrée. Here is the Fat Flush version of fried fish (see following page). I served this to my nephews Isaac and Daniel, who are my most honest taste testers. They don't understand what the fuss is all about—it's just fried fish. *One Sweet Tooth.* 🦷

212. A wedge of lemon and a few herbs such as dill and parsley are often the very best condiments for topping fish. It's an added bonus that they just happen to be low in sugars.

CRISPY UNFRIED FISH 🦷

1 egg, beaten

¼ teaspoon ginger

2 slices HealthSeed spelt bread, toasted and processed
in blender for 1 cup bread crumbs

½ teaspoon garlic powder

¼ teaspoon cayenne

¼ teaspoon dry mustard

4 (5-ounce) fish fillets (sole, sea bass, cod)

Juice of 1 lemon

Fresh parsley for garnish

Preheat oven to 475 degrees. In a large bowl, combine the beaten egg and ginger. In another bowl, mix together the bread crumbs, garlic powder, cayenne, and dry mustard. Dip each fillet into the egg mixture and then coat it with the seasoned bread crumb mixture. Place the fillets on a nonstick cooking sheet. Bake for about 8 minutes or until fish is golden or cooked through. Squeeze lemon juice over the fish. Garnish with parsley and serve. *Serves 4.* 🦷

213. Eating cold-water fish rich in omega-3 essential fatty acids (EFAs) is good for health in general, but it may be particularly helpful for diabetics. Omega-3 EFAs supplied by fish are believed to increase the efficiency of insulin because some studies show that diabetics who take omega-3 EFAs are able to decrease their dosage of insulin. Although more studies need to be done, I recommend that most of my clients eat cold-water fish rich in omega-3

EFAs at least once a week. Omega-3-rich fish include salmon, tuna, trout, mackerel, sardines, cod, and herring.

* **Bonus Tip** When choosing fish, keep in mind that some fish are not your friends due to high methylmercury levels. While not everyone needs to become a mercury detective, understand that if you are pregnant, are nursing, or are thinking about becoming pregnant, you should avoid fish known to be higher in mercury, including shark, swordfish, king mackerel, and tilefish. The general rule is the larger the fish, the larger the mercury numbers. This does not mean to deny yourself or your baby or young child the benefits of fish, since it is safe to eat about 12 ounces per week of cooked, low-mercury fish such as salmon, pollock, catfish, shrimp, and canned light tuna (albacore tuna is higher in mercury than canned light tuna, so don't eat more than 6 ounces per week).

214. **Convenient frozen fish products** to have on hand when you don't want to cook are Salmon Medallions, Halibut Medallions, and Tuna-Pesto Medallions from Northwest Naturals. (They're all sugar-free.)

215. **And what could be more convenient than canned tuna?** Open up a can for a meal anytime, anywhere, for a great source of blood-sugar-stabilizing protein.

216. **Don't forget about shellfish** such as shrimp and scallops. They are powerhouses of minerals, such as zinc, that are balancing to the blood sugar.

points to ponder about pasta

217. **You've heard by now: If you've been piling the pasta on your plate** in an effort to get the fat out of your diet and off your body, you are actually sabotaging your effort.

218. **Don't forget that the commercial pasta** you buy in supermarkets and get in restaurants is made from wheat that has had most of its nutrients stripped away. Although it has some B vitamins and iron added back in, white pasta is missing all the other nutrients important for proper blood sugar function—especially chromium, manganese, and zinc.

219. **Try not to make pasta the cornerstone of your meal.** Use it as a side dish instead, and replace white pasta with the whole-grain variety. Whole-grain spaghetti still raises the blood sugar more than whole grains do (because it's more processed than whole grains), but its higher nutrient and fiber content makes it a much better choice for your blood sugar and your health than white pasta.

220. **If you don't like whole-wheat spaghetti,** try brown rice spaghetti, a mild, versatile, whole-grain pasta that's

better liked than whole-wheat spaghetti by people who are used to refined pasta.

221. **Or try pasta made from spelt,** an unusual-sounding grain that is regarded as a delicacy in Germany and other parts of Europe. With its pleasant, almost nutty flavor, spelt pasta is a well-loved, nutritious addition to the diets of people who have come to realize that white pasta is not in the best interests of their blood sugar. If you'd like to try spelt pasta, look for an assortment of pasta shapes and sizes by Vita-Spelt.

222. **As the name implies, spaghetti squash is a perfect substitute for spaghetti.** The next time you make an Italian pasta or pesto sauce, try using baked spaghetti squash in place of pasta. To make enough for four main-course entrées or six side dishes, follow my easy squash recipe.

BAKED SPAGHETTI SQUASH 🦷

1 large or 2 small spaghetti squash
Italian tomato sauce or pesto sauce

Deeply pierce the skin of the squash in several places with a fork and place in a baking dish. Preheat oven to 375 degrees and bake the squash for 25 minutes, or until the skin is soft to the touch. Let the squash cool for 10 minutes, then cut in half lengthwise. With a spoon, remove the seeds and strings from the center of the squash, then fluff up the flesh with 2 forks until you have spaghettilike strands. Transfer to serving plates and top with sauce. *Makes 4 main course servings or 6 side dish servings.* 🦷

223. Or use steamed shredded zucchini in place of pasta.

amber waves of grains and beans

224. When eaten in moderation, unrefined whole grains can go a long way toward balancing your blood sugar. Don't forget that complex carbohydrates such as these release their sugars slowly and gradually in the system, the way that is best for your sugar-handling mechanisms. In addition, whole grains that have their bran and germ intact are chock-full of blood-sugar-regulating nutrients and fiber.

225. Use brown rice instead of white rice. Brown rice has such a delightful flavor and chewy texture that most people wonder why they ever ate white rice to begin with. To make it, add 2 cups of water or stock and 1 cup of brown rice in a saucepan, heat it to a boil, then turn the heat down and let it simmer for 40–50 minutes (usually 40 minutes for short-grain and 50 minutes for long-grain).

226. If you live life in the fast lane, use quick-cooking brown rice. It's a snap to make, and it's becoming available from several different companies. Two brands I like are

Arrowhead Mills Instant Brown Rice and Lundberg Farms
Quick Brown Rice.

227. **Try other whole grains for variety.** All are packed with
nutrition, and each one has a special taste all its own. If
you're not familiar with whole grains, here are a few you
should get to know:

Brown basmati rice: a type of brown rice that has a
delightful popcorn-like aroma and is particularly good
in Indian dishes.

Barley: a chewy whole grain used primarily in soups,
but it's delicious as a side dish for beef and lamb
dishes as well.

Millet: a gluten-free grain that has a pleasant, slightly
nutty flavor.

Quinoa: a strange-sounding food (pronounced "keen-
wa") that's not in the grain family but is often called a
supergrain because it's packed with nutrition and is a
complete source of protein all on its own. Its light
flavor goes well in soups, salads, and pilafs.

228. **Legumes such as beans and peas are not only
low in fat,** they're low on the glycemic index as well.

> ✳ ***Bonus Tip*** If you haven't eaten many beans before, try
> soaking dry beans overnight before cooking to make them
> more digestible, and start out eating small portions.

Although most legumes contain some naturally occurring sugars, they cause only a minimal rise in blood sugar. This is just one more reason you should eat them.

229. **Blackstrap molasses is high in nutrients and sweetening power,** so a little bit in such dishes as sweet beans is all you need. The following recipe, from *Healing with Whole Foods* by Paul Pitchford, demonstrates this. *One Sweet Tooth.* 🦷

BAKED SWEET BEANS 🦷

2 cups soaked beans (adzuki, lima, navy, or kidney)
8 cups water
½ onion, chopped (optional)
1 tablespoon molasses
1 teaspoon dry mustard
¼–½ teaspoon salt

Discard soaking water and place soaked legumes in a pot with fresh cold water. Place pot on top of the stove. Bring to a boil for 15 minutes to loosen skins. Pour legumes and water into a baking dish. Cover and place in a 350-degree oven for 3–4 hours. When beans are about 80 percent done, add the rest of the ingredients. Then return to oven and cook until soft. Remove the cover to brown. *Serves 6 to 8.* 🦷

vegetables side and center

230. **"Have you had your vegetables today?"** That's a question you should ask yourself each and every day. High in antioxidants and fiber, vegetables are also low in sugars, fat, and calories. They're what nutritionists call "nutrient-dense foods." What more could you ask for? Eat them liberally, three to five times daily.

231. **Vegetables that are fresh and in season** taste great and don't cry out for seasoning of any kind, let alone some type of sweet sauce. Try growing your own or shopping in farmers' markets if you're so inclined, and buy organically grown produce when available. You're likely to taste the difference.

232. **Vary the veggies you eat** to keep your diet interesting. This is always important, but especially when your diet becomes more limited because you're avoiding sugar-rich foods. Actually, you should look at your new eating plan this way: When you get the sugar out of your diet, you're not so much giving up some kinds of foods as you are making room for more essential ones—such as vegetables.

233. **With or without meat,** stir-fried vegetables are a great (sugar-free) way to get even the staunchest vegetable avoiders to eat their veggies.

234. **Chinese five-spice powder, with its sweet, licorice-like taste,** is a delightful way to sweeten any stir-fry. Here's one delicious example from my book *Beyond Pritikin*.

FIVE-SPICE CHICKEN AND
VEGETABLE SAUTÉ 🦷

½ cup chicken broth
2 whole chicken breasts (2 pounds total), skinned, boned,
and cut into ½-inch pieces
2 stalks broccoli, diagonally sliced and lightly steamed
½ red bell pepper, sliced
2 carrots, diagonally sliced and lightly steamed
2 yellow crookneck squash, diagonally sliced (optional)
¼ cup sliced onion
¼ cup canned water chestnuts, drained and sliced
1 tablespoon chopped fresh parsley
¼ teaspoon Chinese five-spice powder
2 cups cooked brown rice

Heat chicken broth in a skillet or wok. Add chicken and cook until tender. Remove chicken from broth and set aside. Add broccoli, red bell pepper, carrots, squash, onion, and water chestnuts. Cook, stirring, 2 to 3 minutes. Add parsley, five-spice powder, and brown rice. Return cooked chicken to mixture. Stir until thoroughly heated. *Serves 4.* 🦷

235. **If heating up a TV dinner is more your style** than cooking a vegetarian meal from scratch, you're in luck. Several companies now offer vegetarian frozen entrées such as lasagna, enchiladas, and macaroni and cheese that don't contain added sugar. Brands to look for include Amy's and Cedarlane, and Taj of India makes good vegetarian Indian entrées.

236. **A cooked sweet potato** is a great way to satisfy your sweet tooth. Full of fiber and nutrients, sweet potatoes also have another unexpected advantage: They rank only 48 on the glycemic index. That means you can enjoy their special sweet flavor without experiencing a drastic rise in your blood sugar.

237. **Here's some news that probably sounds too good to be true:** Eating your baked potato with a little butter, high-quality oil, sour cream, or low-fat cheese is better for your blood sugar than eating it plain. This tip might go against everything you've been led to believe, but here are the facts: A baked potato is a very high inducer of insulin. It ranks between 80 and 89 on the glycemic index. But eating fat or protein with that potato will slow down the insulin response and keep your blood sugar steadier.

238. **Eating sulfur-rich onions** may be normalizing to the blood sugar and especially good for diabetics. In studies in Israel, the sulfur-containing component in onion was found to lower blood sugar and raise the levels of insulin in the cells. For this reason, I recommend using onions often in such dishes as stir-fries, soups, and stews. Or try baking one for a delicious, simple side dish (see following page).

239. **Good things sometimes come in small, unexpected packages.** Such is the case with the little-used vegetable the Jerusalem artichoke. Also called sunchoke, this small, sweet, tuber-like vegetable contains naturally occurring FOS (see tip 71) and is a unique source of inulin, a hormone-like chemical

that reduces insulin needs and may be particularly beneficial for diabetics. If you'd like to try Jerusalem artichokes, eat them raw by themselves, spread them with nut butter, or dip them in a dressing. You can also lightly stir-fry them with other vegetables or sauté them in a garlic-herb butter.

BAKED SWEET ONION

1 large Spanish onion (or Walla Walla, Vidalia,
or Maui, if available)

Keep the skin on the onion intact. Place in a baking pan and bake at 400 degrees for 1 hour. To serve, remove the outer skin and slice off the root end. *Serves 1.*

240. **Get to know the low-starch vegetables,** those that raise the blood sugar only slightly. If you are having trouble maintaining a balanced blood sugar or your proper weight, it may help to emphasize lean meats and the following low-starch vegetables: asparagus, green beans, wax beans, broccoli, Brussels sprouts, cabbage, cauliflower, celery, cucumbers, endive, kale, romaine or leaf lettuce, mushrooms, mustard greens, peppers, radishes, and spinach.

a sauce for all seasons

241. **Sugar- and salt-containing sauces** have a way of covering up the unpleasant taste of processed foods. It's my

hunch that that's why sauces are used so much these days. Be sure to use a sauce on entrées for the right reason: to accentuate the flavor of the whole-food ingredients you're using, not to disguise the taste of lifeless refined foods.

242. **Make the sauce with unrefined foods, too.** Don't make the mistake of cooking fresh meat and fresh vegetables and then covering them up with a gravy made with all-purpose flour. Use a whole-grain flour instead.

> ✱ *Bonus Tip* Powdered arrowroot or kudzu root also work well as thickeners. Dissolve a tablespoon of one of them in liquid and add during the last five minutes of simmering your sauce.

243. **Or use a tablespoon of peanut butter** for a whole new taste. Peanut butter adds more protein and minerals to a sauce than flour does, and also imparts extra richness and creaminess.

244. **Sometimes a little spice is nice.** That's when Indian sauces such as those from Geetha's Gourmet or Taj of India come in handy. With no refined sugar and such varieties as Madras Herb and Bombay Almond, these simmer sauces can quickly transform any plain meat, beans, or vegetables of your choice into Indian cuisine.

245. In Greek tzatziki sauce, cucumber, herbs, and un-sweetened yogurt combine to create a cooling contrast to the spicy beef, lamb, or chicken shish kebabs this sauce usually tops. With no sugar and such simple ingredients, the sauce is delightfully easy to make, too. (See tip 196 for the recipe.)

246. Tabasco hot sauce can splash a little south-of-the-border seasoning on your foods. Containing only cayenne, vine-gar, and salt, Tabasco is a bold seasoning that is partic-ularly good on meats and Mexican dishes, and it's entirely sugar-free.

247. The same holds true for salsa, which is just as good to dab on entrées and side dishes as it is to dip chips in.

248. A dash of tamari (Japanese-style soy sauce) is an easy, sugarless way to give your foods a Chinese flair. Steer clear of teriyaki and sweet-and-sour sauces, though; they're both made with sugar.

249. Pasta sauce can be an unexpected source of sugars. This is surprising because the tomatoes from which pasta sauce is made are naturally sweet. A brand such as Prego may advertise that "it's in there," but I bet you didn't know that meant corn syrup and up to 15 grams of sugars were "in there." Look for a brand that contains no added sugar (such as Muir Glen Garden Vegetable or Portabello Mushroom) or for one that has 5 grams of sugars or less per serving.

250. Or make your own without any added sugar. Holly Sollars, a natural-food recipe tester and developer from Tucson, Arizona, reports that dry-sautéing flavorful vegetables produces a naturally sweet sauce. Besides, pasta sauce always tastes better when it's homemade, anyway. Here's Holly's recipe for Fresh Pasta Sauce that utilizes this helpful tip. *One Sweet Tooth.* 🦷

FRESH PASTA SAUCE 🦷

1½ teaspoons extra-virgin olive oil
1 medium red onion, diced
1 clove garlic, minced
¼ pound mushrooms, sliced thin
2 tablespoons rosé wine (optional)
3–4 medium tomatoes, peeled and diced or pureed
1 15-ounce can organic tomato sauce
1½ tablespoons minced basil (or 2 teaspoons dried)
1½ teaspoons minced oregano (or ¾ teaspoon dried)
Pepper

Heat olive oil in pan, then sauté together the onion, garlic, and mushrooms, stirring constantly, for 1 minute. Add the wine and sauté for 1 or 2 minutes more. Add the tomatoes to the sautéed mixture along with the tomato sauce, basil, oregano, and pepper to taste. Simmer on low, covered, for 30–45 minutes. *Makes about 4 cups.* 🦷

Note: To peel tomatoes, cut an X at the blossom end of each tomato with a paring knife. Core the other end. Place the tomato in boiling water for 30–40 seconds. Remove from the boiling water and place in ice-cold water until cold to the touch. Pull skin off each tomato.

251. **Pesto sauce** is a great example of how sauces made with natural ingredients are truly delectable without sugar of any kind. Made with fresh basil, parsley, nuts, garlic, Parmesan cheese, and olive oil, pesto sauce is great on vegetables, whole-grain pasta, and whole grains such as brown rice. When you don't have time to make this traditional fresh basil sauce at home, use a commercial brand such as Rising Sun Farms to help you make a quick dinner.

252. **My Fat Flush West Indian Seasoning** gives grains and pasta a real kick. If you like it hot, this really spices up seafood, meats, and poultry, too. You can make this up fresh weekly and change the ingredients for more or less heat. *One Sweet Tooth.* 🦷

FAT FLUSH WEST INDIAN SEASONING 🦷

4 scallions, chopped
½ cup fresh lime juice
½ cup finely chopped parsley
1 garlic clove, minced
2 small jalapeños, seeded and minced
1 teaspoon cayenne

Place all ingredients in a food processor or blender. Process until finely chopped. Transfer to a storage container, cover, and refrigerate. *Yields about 1 cup.* 🦷

253. **A few tablespoons of barbecue sauce** can make a sugar-free entrée of fish, meat, or fowl suddenly turn into the sugar equivalent of a heavily sweetened dessert. Whether they're sweetened with sugar, brown sugar, corn syrup, honey, molasses, or fruit juice, commercial barbecue sauces are just too sweet to recommend in their straight form. If you must buy a commercial sauce, check the labels and look for the lowest-sugar version you can find. Then lower its sugar content even more by diluting it with water before using on your food.

254. **Or make my healthy barbecue sauce** from *The Fat Flush Cookbook. One Sweet Tooth.* 🦷

HEALTHY BARBECUE SAUCE 🦷

½ cup finely chopped onion
2 garlic cloves, minced
2 tablespoons plus ¼ cup beef broth
¼ cup apple cider vinegar
1 teaspoon onion powder
½ teaspoon Stevia Plus
1 8-ounce can no-salt-added Muir Glen Tomato Puree
1 teaspoon cayenne, or to taste
½ jalapeño, seeded and minced

Sauté onion and garlic in 2 tablespoons broth until tender. Add remaining broth, vinegar, onion powder, Stevia Plus, tomato puree, cayenne, and jalapeño. Bring to a boil, reduce heat, and simmer for about 30 minutes. Cool and store in the fridge. *Yields about 1 cup.* 🦷

chapter 5

get the sugar out of sandwiches and snacks

Sandwich fixings, condiments, and snacks offer the ultimate in convenience—little fuss, little preparation time, and food at our fingertips.

The quick simplicity of these products sometimes sounds too good to be true—and it is. We're paying a price for these packaged products in the form of hidden sugars, which add up in calories (and, eventually, in excess weight).

At first glance, the sugar content of cold cuts, condiments, and easy-to-grab snack foods doesn't seem like that big a deal. But a gram of sugar here and a few grams of sugar there eventually add up. Before you know it, you consume as much sugar (and calories) in one serving of snack foods as you do eating a rich, sugary dessert. Little by little, day after day, these seemingly insignificant sugar sources increase in number and take their toll on our overworked sugar-balancing systems.

Getting the sugar out of sandwiches and snacks does not mean the end of convenience. Some easy-to-use commercial products fit nicely into a low-sugar way of life, and this chapter will point them out. Also, some recipes (such as the one for Fat Flush Petite Pizzas in tip 272) can be ultimate time savers. If you make a batch of these and freeze them, you have truly fast food that's both nutritious and low in sugars.

Last, remember that you get a great bonus when you get the sugar out of sandwiches and snacks and use fresh ingredients instead. The taste of these foods measurably improves and becomes much more satisfying.

sandwich fixings

255. **High-quality whole-grain bread** can make your sandwich special. Review the "Breads and Spreads" section in chapter 2 if you need a refresher course on how to pick out this crucial sandwich component.

256. **Steer clear of cold cuts,** those convenient sandwich fillers that have the nasty habit of containing unwanted sugars and additives.

257. **Make sandwiches with slices of leftover roast chicken, turkey, or roast beef,** all of which are sugar-free. Finish your sandwich off with red onion slices, red leaf lettuce, and a dab of gourmet mustard and you will have a sandwich fit for a king or queen.

258. **Or use flaked canned tuna** or salmon.

259. **Or try hard-boiled egg slices** and a potpourri of healthy vegetables such as avocado and tomato slices, green pepper strips, and spinach leaves.

260. **Definitely spread your bread with unsweetened peanut butter** (or any other unsweetened nut butter), but skip the jelly. For a real treat, try thin apple or pear slices on your sandwich in place of jelly. *One Sweet Tooth.* 🦷

261. **Mix nut butter with shredded or scraped carrot** for a sandwich filling. *One Sweet Tooth.* 🦷

262. **Bean spreads** are nice vegetarian alternatives to the usual sandwich fare. Watch out for sweetened, fat-free bean spreads, however. Like many other fat-free foods, these products now have sugar in place of fat.

condiments to relish

263. **Choose your condiments with care** and go over those labels with a fine-tooth comb. Small amounts of sugars tend to creep into everything from mayo to relish and gradually add up. Remember, if you have a tablespoon of mayo and a tablespoon of ketchup on your burger, you consume 6 grams of unnecessary sugars. I personally prefer to skip these condiments altogether and occasionally treat myself to a cookie with 6 grams of sugars instead.

• •

264. **Hold the salt** for a couple of reasons. First, too much salt in the diet can cause sugar cravings (as explained in tip 36). Second, commercial salt contains dextrose, which is another crafty way of saying sugar.

265. **Understand that salt and sugar tend to go hand in hand in condiments.** The more manufacturers add of one, the more they add of the other—and our taste buds lose track of how much of both of them we taste. This is why many condiments, such as ketchup and barbecue sauce, contain more sugar than some desserts but we don't perceive them as being that sweet.

266. **Pass up the commercial ketchup,** a little something that seems so innocent but is really a sugar monger in disguise. In every tablespoon of ketchup, you get a whole teaspoon of sugar. In fact, ounce for ounce, ketchup has more sugar in it than ice cream!

267. **If your meal won't be complete without your favorite red spread,** seek out Westbrae Natural Unsweetened Un-Ketchup. Feel free to use a tablespoon of this ketchup on burgers and such without guilt. It's sugar-free. *One Sweet Tooth.* 🦷

268. **Become a mustard connoisseur.** Whether you use regular, stone-ground, Dijon-style, or horseradish-spiked, mustard is one condiment that is almost always sugarless. Have fun experimenting with different varieties of this pungent spread in a variety of ways. (It goes without saying, how-

ever, that you should continue to read the labels of the
mustards you buy. You never know when manufacturers
might decide to add sugar.)

269. **When a tablespoon of mayonnaise is what your
sandwich needs,** make sure to use a brand, such as Spectrum Naturals, that contains no refined sugar. Try either
Spectrum's Canola Mayonnaise, which is sweetened with
honey and contains only 1 gram of sugar per tablespoon,
or its Light Canola Mayo, which is sugar-free. *One Sweet
Tooth.*

270. **Or make your sandwich Italian-style.** Dress it with
oregano and a vinegar-and-oil dressing for a new approach
to your usual lunch.

the snack cart

271. **Avoid eating sweets between meals.** Sure, we all get
the munchies, but satisfying this need with sugary snacks is
extremely stressful to the body (not to mention hard on the
teeth). A satisfying snack will tide you over and keep you
alert and energetic until your next meal. In-between-meal
sweets don't meet that definition. Try instead more substantial mini-meals.

272. **A guilt-free pizza snack:** just what the doctor ordered to
keep you satisfied and sugar-free between meals. My Fat
Flush Petite Pizza recipe provides you with one of the

easiest ways to help you get the sugar out of your diet in between meals because it offers satisfying smart carbs and just the right amount of fat to keep your blood sugar stable. If you have a supply of these in your freezer, you have complete, ready-to-eat, sugar-free meals at your fingertips—good for snacking or for breakfasts or lunch on the run. *One Sweet Tooth.* 🦷

FAT FLUSH PETITE PIZZA 🦷

1 slice HealthSeed spelt bread, toasted
Pinch dried oregano
4 tablespoons no-salt-added tomato sauce
Pinch garlic powder
Pinch ground fennel
1 ounce shredded part-skim mozzarella cheese

Preheat oven to 300 degrees. Place bread on nonstick cookie sheet. Add oregano to tomato sauce and spread on bread. Sprinkle with garlic powder and fennel. Add cheese. Bake for about 8 minutes or until cheese is melted. *Serves 1.* 🦷

273. **Try low-fat cheese on whole-grain crackers** such as whole-wheat matzo or such Scandinavian flatbreads as Kavli or Ryvita.

274. **Have some vegetable "chips" and dip.** Cut up vegetables such as carrots, celery, jicama, and green pepper into stick or chip shapes and serve with a low-sugar dip such as

the Greek Tzatziki Sauce in tip 196 or the Avocado Cilantro Dip in tip 294.

275. **Spread celery with nut butter** for a quick, crunchy treat.

276. **Unsweetened bean spreads** go well on whole-grain tortillas or chapatis.

277. **Half a turkey or tuna sandwich**—on whole-grain bread, of course—makes a great snack.

278. **Improvise a mini-meal from leftovers.** Here's one example: Reheat leftover brown rice, coat it with sesame or sunflower butter, and top with a few pieces of chopped dried fruit and a dash of cinnamon. *One Sweet Tooth.* 🦷

279. **Nuts are a natural for nibbling,** but be careful which types you consume. The honey-roasted varieties obviously are high in sugar, but did you know that sugar is often used in dry-roasting as well? If you've been eating dry-roasted nuts to lessen your fat intake, you've probably been eating hidden sugar instead. Here's a way to avoid extra fat and sugar by home-toasting raw nuts. Simply spread shelled raw nuts of your choice on a cookie sheet and bake at 275 degrees for 5–15 minutes (depending on the size of the nuts). The nuts are both nutritious and delicious.

280. **Low-sugar granola or granola bars can be satisfying,** but be especially careful with this suggestion. Most

granola products on the market are cookies disguised as health food. The homemade granola in tip 150 and the granola bar below, however, are delicious exceptions that can work nicely as snacks or for on-the-go breakfasts. *One Sweet Tooth.* 🦷

ALMOND-OAT SQUARES 🦷

2 cups rolled oats
½ cup chopped or sliced almonds
¼ cup oat bran
¼ cup sesame seeds
Pinch salt (optional)
⅔ cup applesauce or mashed banana
⅔ cup almond butter, room temperature

Combine the oats, almonds, bran, sesame seeds, and salt in a large bowl. In a small bowl, mix together the applesauce or mashed banana and the almond butter until well blended. Scrape the almond butter mixture into the oat mixture, mix well, then pat into an 11-by-7-inch baking dish. Bake at 300 degrees for about 35 minutes. Score with a knife while warm, then cut into square or bar shapes when cool. *Serves 4.* 🦷

Variation: Use chopped peanuts and peanut butter or chopped cashews and cashew butter in place of the almonds and almond butter.

281. Ground flaxseeds pack a nutritional punch that is not only high in fiber but high in heart-healthy

omega-3s. This recipe comes from my book *The Fast Track Detox Diet. One Sweet Tooth.* 🦷

SWEETIE PIE FLAX SNACK CRACKERS 🦷

½ cup ground flaxseeds
2 teaspoons ground cinnamon
½ teaspoon ground cloves
1 teaspoon whey protein powder
Dash powdered stevia
1 teaspoon ground allspice

Preheat the oven to 250 degrees. Spray a cookie sheet with olive oil spray. Mix the flaxseeds, cinnamon, cloves, whey protein powder, stevia, and allspice together. Add enough filtered water (about ¼ cup) to form the mixture into a ball. Place the dough between two pieces of wax paper. Roll very thin. Remove the paper, transfer the dough to the cookie sheet, and score the dough into 2-inch-square crackers. Bake 30 to 40 minutes, until the crackers pull up from the cookie sheet. Store in a cool place. *Makes 36 crackers.* 🦷

chapter 6

get the sugar out of drinks and party foods

most people seem to forget that beverages are part of their diets, too. Even when they watch their diets carefully, many Americans will think nothing of having a large glass of juice with breakfast, a can of cola with lunch and for a snack, and an alcoholic drink with dinner. They fail to realize that these liquids alone can easily add up to 125 grams of sugars—well over the amount that is known to significantly impair the immune system. They also forget that these drinks will add an extra 500 calories a day to their tally, very likely adding an extra pound of fat to their body each week.

Drinks certainly don't have to add weight, though. They can be refreshing, thirst-quenching, and even slightly sweet without being significant sources of sugars and calories. The tips in this chapter will point you toward ways to get the sugar out of the drinks you consume, but the first thing to remember is that good old sugar-free water is the best thirst quencher of all. Our bodies are more than two-thirds water, and every fluid and tissue that we have, from our blood to our bones, requires water to function properly. It's vital to understand that water is the only drink that's a nutrient all by itself—and something we should all drink more of. If you can make only one change in your diet, switching from drinking sugary soda to purified water will get significant sugar out of your diet and is one of the most health-promoting changes I can recommend.

Unlike beverages that we consume every day, party foods are reserved for special occasions. From what I've seen in my clients' food diaries, these special occasions often turn into sugary occasions. Hidden in some of the most basic party hors d'oeuvres and entrées are sugars galore, and the sugar grams escalate to hazardous levels when typical party and holiday desserts are served.

You don't have to be a party pooper or holiday Scrooge by serving less sweet food. To have your guests raving, use the freshest ingredients possible combined with irresistible herbs in the hors d'oeuvres and entrées you serve. Your guests' taste buds will be so tantalized that no one will miss the sugar. Then, if you want to have a sweet end to your event, by all means serve a dessert—just make sure it's a healthy one.

As I see it, drinks and party foods are extras in life. If we neglect to choose with care the ones we consume, they can be significant sources of extra calories that put on extra weight. But if we know how to get the sugar out of them, drinks and party foods can be additional sources of health-promoting nutrients as well as special treats.

drinking to health

282. If you do nothing else to get the sugar out of your diet, just get the sugar out of the beverages you consume. Drinks are such common sources of empty calories that they are usually the first area I look at when I'm counseling my clients.

283. Begin by steering clear of soft drinks, the greatest single contributor of sugar in our diets. (This is an obvious tip that you should know by now!) Soft drinks are harmful to your health in every way, shape, and form, whether you're talking about the 39 grams of sugars in one can of Coke, the phosphoric acid that throws your calcium balance out of whack, or the caffeine that continually stresses

---

* Bonus Tip If you just can't seem to give up your soda, there is good news; you can finally just say no—no sugar, no carbs, no artificial sweeteners, no caffeine, no calories, no preservatives, no sodium, no dairy, no gluten, and no GMOs. Yes, the first natural diet soda in America is now being made by a company called Sulo, which makes their sodas with stevia instead of sugar or aspartame. To find out where Sulo Healthy Soda Natural Diet Cola and Natural Diet Ginger Ale are available in your area, call 828-253-2663 or 877-810-0696, or visit www.suloinc.com.

your adrenal glands. As the authors of *Eating for A's* said in their book, the sugar content of soft drinks makes them nothing more than "liquid candy bars with fizz."

284. Diet drinks are dangerous and definite no-nos even when you're trying to avoid sugar. (See tips 48–58 for more explanation.) Not only are aspartame-sweetened drinks believed to deplete the body of chromium, a mineral important for proper blood sugar functioning, but storing these drinks in a hot place may cause the aspartame in them to break down into toxic chemicals that can cause a multitude of health problems. Many still believe that Desert Storm syndrome, an unexplained illness that affected thousands of Desert Storm soldiers, may have been caused by this phenomenon.

285. The easiest substitute for soda is juice mixed with sparkling mineral water. This drink still contains natural sugars, but it has less sugar than soft drinks and certainly more vitamins and minerals. Watch out for premade juice-and-sparkling-water combinations, though. Many of these drinks appear healthful but actually include sugar and high-fructose corn syrup, which turn the drinks into high-priced sodas. Far better for you to make this drink yourself so you can control the amount of sugar you ingest. Usually *Two Sweet Teeth.* 🦷🦷

286. Homemade ginger ale is not only more tasty, more nutritious, and far lower in sugar than most commercial

consumer alert
THE 411 ON BOTTLED H$_2$O

There is no doubt about it: bottled water is here to stay. In 2006 U.S. bottled water sales reached $9 billion dollars—giving soda sales a run for the money. (Actually, soda companies also now sell their own brands of bottled water—Coke offers Dasani, Pepsi offers Aquafina.) What was once hailed as the ultimate marketing marvel is now a national mainstay. But are bottled "health waters" really healthy? Is the bottled water phenomenon a convenient way to get your eight glasses of water a day with added taste and even added vitamins and minerals, or is it another source of hidden sugars? Before you fill your fridge, let's take a closer look at bottled H$_2$O.

Is bottled water regulated?
Yes. The FDA describes bottled water as water that is intended for human consumption and that is sealed in bottles or other containers with no added ingredients, except that it may contain a safe and suitable antimicrobial agent. The FDA has set standards for spring, well, mineral, artesian, and purified water. Water that adds flavor, enhancements, or vitamins is considered a soft drink. (Note that the FDA makes adding fluoride optional.) For additional information, contact the Food and Drug Administration, Office of Plant and Dairy Foods and Beverages (HFS-306), 200 C Street, S.W., Washington, D.C. 20204, 202-205-4681.

What's in a name?

• *Spring water* must come from a spring.

• *Well water* comes from a hole bored or drilled into the ground, which taps into an aquifer—layers of porous rock, sand, and earth that contain water.

• *Mineral water* is water from an underground source that contains at least 250 parts per million total dissolved solids. Note that the minerals and trace elements must come from the source of the underground water and cannot be an additive.

• *Artesian well water* must be water from a well that taps a pressurized underground water supply.

• *Purified water* is water that has been treated by distillation, reverse osmosis, or other suitable process to meet the definition of "purified water" in the U.S. Pharmacopeia. There is a pretty good chance that this bottle contains filtered tap water. Did you know that many cities make big money selling their public water supply in bottles under catchy names? The lesson here is you can save money and still have the on-the-go convenience of bottled water by investing in an at-home water filtration system (in the fridge, on the tap, or a whole-house system). Plus by reusing bottles you are also saving the environment.

• *Enhanced and flavored water* can contain anything from vitamin C to skin conditioners and of course sweeteners. Let's face it—the list of flavored waters with way too much sugar is simply too long to include in this book: Instead I will remind you to be a savvy consumer and check the label,

(continued)

since many of those sweet-sounding names can contain as much as 35 grams of sugar per bottle. There are companies that are making the most of the bottled water phenomenon in ways that are innovative without the sugar coating.

• *Borba* water combines hydration with skin care, and while it does contain 1 gram of sugar, it also fortifies the skin with additives such as lychee for hydrating and pomegranate for clarifying. Borba claims to improve skin quality within seven days by providing vitamins and antioxidants from the inside out. Borba Skin Balance Waters are available in Clarifying, Age Defying, Replenishing, Firming, Anti Aging, and Skin Calming. Check out www.borba.net.

• *Trinity* water contains no calories, no carbs, no sugar, and no artificial ingredients of any kind. Trinity comes from what the company claims is world's deepest natural water source, a reservoir in Paradise, Idaho, that lies 2.2 miles below the earth's surface and was last exposed to the atmosphere more than 16,000 years ago. Surrounding granite naturally provides the water with minerals such as fluoride and silica. The high pH of the water, 9.6, makes it alkaline, which may be helpful for those who want to counteract the effects of an acidic diet. For those of you who need a little flavor, *Trinity Organic* adds organic flavors—Lemon, Mint Leaf, Raspberry, Orange Tangerine, Peach Mango, and Coconut. Check out www.trinitysprings.com.

ginger ales, but it's also a snap to make with the help of a wholesome product called Ginger Wonder Syrup by New Moon Extracts. Developed by master herbalist Paul Schulick, Ginger Wonder Syrup contains only pure Vermont honey and juiced, dried, and macerated organic ginger. A highly regarded tonic herb, ginger has natural anti-inflammatory properties, is good for digestive upset, and may in fact have blood-sugar-balancing properties. To make this healthful alternative to soda, just mix 1 teaspoon or less of Ginger Wonder Syrup in 4 ounces of sparkling mineral water. What could be simpler? Look for this product in your local health food store, point your browser to www.newchapter.info, or call 800-543-7279.

287. Use stevia to make great-tasting sweet drinks. My Fat Flush followers rave about the following beverage made with Stevia Plus (see tip 70). They find that this delightful beverage satisfies their need for something sweet without aggravating candidiasis. Here's the refreshing recipe for your enjoyment. *One Sweet Tooth.* 🦷

FAT FLUSH LEMONADE 🦷

¼ cup freshly squeezed lemon juice
¼ teaspoon Stevia Plus or to taste
2 cups purified water, chilled

Combine all ingredients and stir until the Stevia Plus is completely dissolved. Serve cold. *Serves 2.* 🦷

Variation: Substitute lime juice or cranberry juice for the lemon juice.

288. **Make an iced herbal tea.** With so many varieties ranging from fruit-flavored to mint blends, herbal tea can delight just about anyone's taste buds. If you don't like tea plain, try adding just a pinch of the herb stevia or a drop of stevia liquid concentrate to sweeten the tea. *One Sweet Tooth.* 🦷

289. **Another refreshing treat** is to serve sparkling mineral water over ice cubes made from unsweetened natural fruit juices. With this tip you can make colorful drinks that have a touch of fruit sweetness without an excess of sugar. *One Sweet Tooth.* 🦷

290. **Avoid alcohol, which acts like pure sugar in the body** as well as a drug that taxes the liver and causes great nutrient deficiencies and imbalances. Many alcoholics are hypoglycemic, and some doctors now believe that sugar imbalances are a causal factor in alcoholism. It may seem unsocial not to drink alcohol or to drink only occasionally, but it is increasingly accepted and it's one of the simplest things you can do to get the sugar out and maintain good health.

291. **If you do drink alcohol,** make sure to stretch your drink by diluting it with club soda, seltzer, or water and lots of ice. Alcohol acts like sugar and provides empty calories, so moderation is the key here.

292. **Tonic water may seem like a harmless drink,** but don't be fooled. For every 12 ounces of tonic water, you get a whopping 18 teaspoons of sugar! Skip the tonic and start employing the next tip instead.

293. **Sparkling mineral water with a twist of lemon or lime** is your best choice for a sugar-free drink at a cocktail party. Seltzer and club soda also are sugar-free, but many brands of club soda are high in sodium. All of these drinks look so much like a regular alcoholic drink, most people won't know you're not drinking.

---

take a dip

294. **Somehow a party just doesn't seem complete without a good dip** served on a party tray with colorful veggies. Here's a dip that can substitute nicely for the usual ranch dip full of hidden sugars (see following page). *One Sweet Tooth.* 🦷

295. **For an even quicker dip,** use a sugar-free mixing packet such as those from the Spice Hunter. With easy-to-add ingredients and savory herbal combinations, these mixes can make dreamy dips for those who don't have any time to spare.

296. **Salsa, which rarely contains sugar, is a party favorite.** Serve it with strips of cheese-crisp corn tortillas (nachos) for extra fun.

AVOCADO CILANTRO DIP 𝕎

1 large ripe avocado, peeled, pitted, and diced
¼ cup finely chopped scallions
¼ cup chopped fresh cilantro
1 tablespoon fresh lemon juice
2 medium tomatoes, seeded and finely chopped
½ teaspoon ground cumin
1–3 drops hot sauce, such as Tabasco
Salt
1 tablespoon flaxseed oil

Place avocado in a large bowl and mash. Blend in scallions, cilantro, lemon juice, tomatoes, cumin, hot sauce, and salt to taste. Pour in oil and blend, using a wooden spoon. Serve with veggie dippers. *Makes 1 cup.* 𝕎

297. **Don't forget about guacamole,** another Mexican medley of vegetable flavors. If you don't make it from scratch, be sure to buy a brand that doesn't have any added sugars.

298. **Middle Eastern eggplant dip or chickpea-based hummus** are two other sugar-free crowd-pleasers. Serve them with whole-grain pita bread or chapatis.

appetizers and hors d'oeuvres

299. Serve low-fat cheese chunks and hearty whole-grain crackers such as Ryvita Sesame-Rye any time, even for spur-of-the-moment social occasions.

300. Who can resist the smell of freshly made garlic bread? Just about no one that I know of. To make a healthier (but still irresistible) version of this appetizer that's usually made with refined French bread, follow these directions: Mince a few garlic cloves and herbs such as parsley, rosemary, or thyme. Mix the seasonings in 4 tablespoons of soft butter or a combination of butter and olive oil. Spread on top of 10 thick spelt bread or multigrain bread slices and bake at 350 degrees for 10–15 minutes. (Or you can place them under the broiler for a few minutes.) The only word to describe this is *yum*!

301. Barbecued chicken drumsticks or wingdings don't have to be sugar-laden to be gobbled up by your guests. Just use the Healthy Barbecue Sauce from tip 254 on them. You can always kick it up a notch by adding another jalapeño. *One Sweet Tooth.* 🦷

302. Serve barbecued vegetable kebabs with the same sauce. *One Sweet Tooth.* 🦷

303. Or marinate vegetables in a vinaigrette, arrange on kebab skewers, and broil. A few good veggies to include are

pepper and onion chunks, sliced zucchini, whole mushrooms, and cherry tomatoes.

304. **Now here's a marvelous idea for a cocktail party:**
Spinach Stuffed Mushrooms. This is great party food, not
to mention a quick and easy snack for you to pack and take
with you. *One Sweet Tooth.* 🦷

SPINACH-STUFFED MUSHROOMS 🦷

1 10-ounce package frozen spinach, thawed and drained
1 egg yolk
1 garlic clove, minced
12 large white mushrooms, cleaned and stemmed

Heat oven to 350 degrees. Spray a small baking sheet with nonstick cooking spray. In a large bowl, mix spinach, egg yolk, and
garlic. Stuff each mushroom with spinach mixture and place on
baking sheet. Bake for 14–25 minutes or until mixture is firm to
the touch. Serve hot. *Serves 4.* 🦷
Variation: For variety, you can add ½ teaspoon basil and oregano
to the stuffing mix. For another twist, you can add ½ teaspoon
nutmeg and ¼ cup chopped walnuts to the stuffing mix.

305. **Meatballs are versatile hors d'oeuvres** for all occasions. Why are they so versatile? You can make them with
ground turkey, chicken, lamb, or beef—and you can top
them with all kinds of low-sugar sauces ranging from

Swedish-style sauce to pesto sauce to the Pasta Sauce in tip 250. Finally, they're popular with all kinds of people. What more could a host ask for?

306. **Talk about versatile!** Mini shish kebabs certainly fit that description. They can be made with chicken, turkey, lamb, beef, shrimp, scallops, or even a firm fish such as swordfish. To make them, marinate the pieces in a low-sugar salad dressing such as vinaigrette or lemon juice, olive oil, garlic, and oregano. Skewer them on wooden sticks that have been soaked in water for at least 30 minutes, then broil.

> * **Bonus Tip** For the best flavor, marinate meats overnight in the refrigerator. There's no need to do this with seafood and fish, though. They're so delicate that they don't do well with this extra tenderizing.

307. **For an Oriental flair,** make the same shish kebabs but marinate them in tamari combined with sesame oil, fresh ginger, and garlic.

special occasions

308. **A party punch is one of the quickest ways I know of** to consume more sugar than my body can comfortably handle. With ingredients such as sugar, honey, ginger ale,

and fruit juice concentrates, most punches are sugar disasters waiting to happen. This one from *Sweet and Natural* by Janet Warrington isn't, because she cleverly thins out the sugar content of the juices with tea and adds aromatic sweet spices. Good served hot during the holidays or iced during the summer, a 1-cup serving of this punch counts as one fruit exchange on the diabetic food exchange system. *One Sweet Tooth.* 🦷

SPICED TEA 🦷

2½ cups water
3 decaf tea bags (or 3 raspberry-leaf tea bags)
¼ teaspoon ground nutmeg
¼ teaspoon ground cinnamon
2 cups unsweetened apple juice
½ cup unsweetened orange juice
5 orange or lemon slices (optional)

Bring the water to a boil and steep the tea bags and the spices for 3 minutes. Remove the tea bags and stir in the apple juice and orange juice. If serving cold, pour the tea over ice and serve with an orange slice or lemon wedge. If serving hot, bring heat up until the tea simmers, add the orange or lemon wedges, and ladle the tea into mugs. *Serves 5.* 🦷

309. **Festive fruit kebabs** can be served as either a party appetizer or a fun dessert. Arrange a variety of fresh fruit such as pineapple chunks, whole strawberries, banana

slices, and melon balls on wooden skewers and see what a difference innovative food presentation can make. *One Sweet Tooth.* 🦷

310. **Or serve colorful fruit salad** in a watermelon or pineapple boat. This makes an unusually attractive sweet finish to any celebration. *One Sweet Tooth.* 🦷

311. **When a special occasion calls for a special treat,** make sure you use special, high-quality ingredients in place of refined sugar. Here's a good example from *The All-Natural Sugar-Free Dessert Cookbook* by Linda Romanelli Leahy. *Two Sweet Teeth.* 🦷🦷

CHOCOLATE-COATED-FRUIT PARTY PLATTER 🦷🦷

4 ounces unsweetened chocolate
1 tablespoon unsalted butter
½ cup unsweetened apple juice concentrate
1 teaspoon natural vanilla extract
4 cups fresh fruit (whole strawberries, bananas,
navel orange slices, kiwis, etc.)

Spray baking sheet with cooking spray and set aside. In the top of a double boiler, over simmering water, melt chocolate and butter, stirring occasionally; remove from heat and cool slightly. Whisk in juice concentrate a little at a time until chocolate is smooth; add vanilla extract. If mixture is too thick, add a little more concentrate until it thins out. Dip ends of fruit into chocolate mix, twirling to coat lower half of each piece of fruit; let excess drip back into pan until all chocolate is used. Place fruit on prepared baking sheet; place in freezer 10 minutes to set chocolate. Refrigerate until ready to serve. *Makes 12 servings.* 𝅘𝅥 𝅘𝅥

312. Every special summer occasion can use a refreshing splash of color and flavor. This simple yet elegant dip will get your guests talking as it livens up the standard fruit salad. *Three Sweet Teeth.* 𝅘𝅥 𝅘𝅥 𝅘𝅥

REFRESHING SUMMER FRUITS WITH RICOTTA DIP 𝅘𝅥 𝅘𝅥 𝅘𝅥

2 cups ricotta cheese
½ cup plain yogurt
1 tablespoon honey
1 teaspoon vanilla extract
¼ teaspoon cinnamon
4 cups fresh fruit, cut into chunks
(pineapple, berries, melon, etc.)

Combine all the ingredients except the fruit in a blender or food processor; puree until smooth. Pour into a bowl and refrigerate until serving time. Arrange the fruit decoratively around a large plate and place the dip in the center. *Serves 4.* 𝅘𝅥 𝅘𝅥 𝅘𝅥

313. "Have a happy, healthy birthday!" That's what you'll be saying to the guest of honor when you present this wholesome cake instead of the usual store-bought variety. *Two Sweet Teeth.* 🦷🦷

EVERYTHING GOOD BIRTHDAY CAKE 🦷🦷

1½ cups whole-wheat pastry flour
1 teaspoon baking powder
1 teaspoon baking soda
1 teaspoon ground nutmeg
Pinch salt
1 teaspoon ground cinnamon
⅓ cup melted butter or oil
½ cup fruit juice concentrate
2 eggs, beaten
1 cup unsweetened applesauce

Preheat oven to 375 degrees. Combine dry ingredients. In another bowl combine liquid ingredients and add to dry. Mix well. Pour mixture into a 9-inch cake pan and bake for 45 minutes, or until done. Allow to cool. Serve as is or add frosting of your choice from the "Icing on the Cake" section in chapter 7 if desired. *Serves 8 to 10.* 🦷🦷

Note: Beating the egg yolks separately and adding to the wet ingredients, then folding in the beaten egg whites, will produce a fluffier cake.

314. When sugar restriction is necessary for the birthday boy or girl, just ask him or her to pick out the absolute favorite allowable food he or she can eat. Colorful candles can wish just as good tidings on strawberries and whipped cream, a muffin, or even on pizza as they can on a birthday cake, so don't get too tied to tradition. After all, a birthday party is designed to celebrate the person, not the food he or she can eat.

315. **Rethink your attitudes** surrounding birthdays, anniversaries, holidays, and other special occasions. Is it really necessary to have rich, gooey desserts to have a good time? The most festive, happy occasions usually involve just good entertainment and caring family and friends to share in the joyful experience. Don't lose sight of this.

holiday coping strategies

316. *Moderation* **is the key word to keep in mind during the holidays.** Taste the special foods of the season, but don't go overboard. Especially try to avoid indulging in sugary foods during nonsocial occasions.

317. **Eat a protein-rich snack before you go to a party** where you know there will be lots of tempting desserts. A few pieces of chicken or turkey meat beforehand can keep you from being famished at the party and bingeing on too much sugar.

318. **If tired and stressed out is how you usually feel** during the holiday season, avoid eating sweets and keep the

meals that you make simple. Having ready-to-heat left-overs and sugar-free snacks on hand always helps.

319. **Continue to eat well-balanced meals and snacks** during the holidays. Doing so will balance your blood sugar and make you less likely to overindulge in holiday sweets.

320. **When you go on a long holiday shopping spree,** take high-protein snacks with you to sustain you. They'll keep you away from quick-fix sweets sold in shopping-mall food courts. Some good snacks to take are the Peanut Butter Muffins in tip 120, the Fat Flush Petite Pizza in tip 272, or the Almond-Oat Squares in tip 280. Nuts are also good foods to carry along.

321. **Revise your typical holiday meal to lower its sugar content,** and be sure to substitute unrefined grain products for refined carbohydrates. Go ahead and enjoy a serving of stuffing—just make sure it's made with whole grains or whole-grain bread instead of white bread.

322. **To replace sugar-rich canned cranberry sauce,** make this tangy, easy-to-fix, homemade version that's far superior in flavor. This seems like such a natural for Banana French Toast (tip 121)—especially when you have no time to cook. *Two Sweet Teeth.* 🦷 🦷

QUICK CRAN-RASPBERRY SAUCE 🦷🦷

½ cup fresh or frozen cranberries, thawed
½ cup raspberries
½ teaspoon orange zest
¾ teaspoon Stevia Plus

Place all ingredients in a blender and blend until smooth. Heat in a saucepan for about 2 minutes or until hot. *Serves 1.* 🦷🦷

323. **Candied sweet potatoes may be traditional,** but it's silly (and unhealthy) to add loads of concentrated, refined sweeteners to an already perfectly sweet food. Make this subtly sweet basic Sweet Potato Casserole instead for the holidays and everyone will leave satisfied. *One Sweet Tooth.* 🦷

SWEET POTATO CASSEROLE 🦷

6 large sweet potatoes
1 20-ounce can crushed pineapple packed in juice
1 teaspoon ground cinnamon (optional)
1–3 tablespoons sesame oil (optional)
½ cup chopped pecans (optional)

Bake sweet potatoes on a cookie sheet at 375 degrees for about an hour, until done. Cut in half and scoop out the potato flesh. Discard the skin. Mash sweet potato with masher or with an electric mixer on low until smooth. Add pineapple, its juice, the cinnamon, and oil, and mix well. Spoon mixture into a lightly oiled casserole or a 9-by-13-inch baking dish. Sprinkle pecans on top if desired. Cover and bake for about 40 minutes. *Serves 10 to 12.* 𝅘

324. **If you have a traditional holiday recipe** that's been handed down through the ages, feel free to use it as long as you substitute Sucanat, date "sugar," or rice syrup powder in place of the sugar the recipe may call for. (We know the facts about refined sugar better than they did in the good old days.)

325. **Pumpkin pie doesn't have to be terribly sweet to be pleasing.** This recipe will show you what I mean. *Three Sweet Teeth.* 𝅘 𝅘 𝅘

MY PUMPKIN PIE 𝅘𝅘𝅘

1½ cups pumpkin puree
1 teaspoon ground cinnamon
½ teaspoon ground ginger
½ teaspoon ground nutmeg
½ teaspoon ground cloves
3 eggs, beaten
2 tablespoons Fat Flush Vanilla Whey
1 cup water
3 packets Stevia Plus
1 tablespoon molasses
2 tablespoons honey
1 teaspoon vanilla extract
1 whole-grain piecrust

Preheat oven to 425 degrees. Mix pumpkin puree, cinnamon, ginger, nutmeg, and cloves, then stir in beaten eggs. In a large bowl, mix together whey and water. Add to pumpkin-egg mixture. Add Stevia Plus, molasses, honey, and vanilla. Pour filling into crust and bake for 15 minutes at 425 degrees. Reduce heat to 350 degrees and bake for 45–50 minutes longer, or until a knife inserted in the center comes out clean. Cool on wire rack before serving. *Serves 8 to 10.* 🦷 🦷 🦷

326. **Don't give refined, sugary sweets as gifts,** and ask the same of others.

327. **Keep the spirit of the season.** Don't be so hung up on the foods and sweets of the season that you forget to enjoy what's most important: celebrating sweet, memorable times with those you love.

get the sugar out of baking, desserts, and treats

*m*y work with clients for more than twenty-five years has led me to conclude that most Americans fall into one of four types of dessert eaters—and none of these really knows how to get the sugar out of their diet.

Type one is what I call the traditional dessert eater. This type indulges in desserts with a high fat and high refined-sugar content—foods such as cream pies, rich fudge, and butter cookies. The high fat content of these desserts is extremely satisfying and filling for traditional dessert eaters, but even the high fat content can't keep their excessive sugar consumption from taxing their blood-sugar-balancing mechanisms and causing them harm.

The second type is the natural-goodie dessert eater, also sometimes known as the health buff. This kind will eat anything as long as it's made with natural sweeteners and whole-grain flours.

Health buffs are correct in part of their dessert philosophy—it is far better to consume goodies made with unrefined sweeteners and whole grains rather than those made with processed carbohydrates. Unfortunately, health buffs have conveniently forgotten about an equally important component of maintaining health—keeping the sugars one consumes, even the natural sugars, to an absolute minimum.

Type three is the fat-free-goodie eater. Americans have gotten some ill-conceived advice about fat in the past, and in a misguided attempt to avoid all fat, we are consuming more sugars than ever before, missing out on an essential nutrient (fat) that could help moderate our blood-sugar levels. As a result, people are pigging out on fat-free foods they think are good for them and yet wondering why they are so tired, overweight, and disease-prone.

Type four is the carb-counting dessert eater who will eat just about anything as long as it is low in carbs. As a result, these individuals may be not only omitting necessary good carbs but are making themselves cranky, forgetful, and depressed. A balanced diet should include the healthy carbs that can be found in whole fruits, root vegetables, whole grains, and legumes along with eggs, turkey, and a modified intake of dairy products. These foods help your body to produce serotonin, a brain chemical that produces a state of comfort, calm, and alertness. Low-carb diets that produce insufficient amounts of serotonin contribute to depression, sleeplessness, migraine, PMS, and impulsive behavior, including binge eating. Low serotonin levels make it hard to say no at the same time that they create even more of a craving for carbs and sweets in a misguided attempt to balance out their nutritional imbalance.

Although these four types of dessert eaters seem vastly different, they share one common bond—they want to feel good and look good. They all need to learn that moderation and balance among all nutrients is the key to healthy and enjoyable dessert eating. Most important, we all need to understand that the more we can cut down on sugars in the treats we consume, the better off our health will be.

Switching from enjoying a piece of cake with 25 grams of sugars to one with 5 grams is like going from *A* to *Z*. I wouldn't be honest or fair if I told you that you can make the switch overnight. You cannot. It has taken years for you to get used to the amount of sugars you currently consume in sweets, so be patient with yourself and realize that it's going to take a while to wean yourself away from all those sugars and to retrain your sweet tooth.

The tips in this chapter will show you practical ways to reduce the amount of sugars in the treats you buy and make. But overly sweetened desserts will forever tempt you until you develop a firm resolve about how vitally important it is to lower your sugar intake. If you start to forget just why you were getting the sugar out of your diet, copy the list of health problems associated with excessive sugar intake from pages 26–27 and put it up on your refrigerator. This should be an effective reminder of how much you need to consciously and persistently work at reducing your sugar intake each and every day—even in the desserts you consume.

Despite what you might believe, getting the sugar out of sweet treats does not mean eating tasteless desserts. I think you will be amazed at just how satisfying and special some of the minimally sweetened desserts in this section really are.

Even if some of the One Sweet Tooth–designated desserts

initially seem too bland for your taste buds, you will be surprised at how much your taste buds can change. If you continue to eat less sugary foods, you will gradually but honestly come to prefer them, just as I have.

Treats are special simply because they are not something you have every day. But when you get the sugar out of the other areas of your diet, you may find that you can treat yourself a little more often to sweet indulgences as long as they are subtly sweetened, nutritionally balanced, and made with wholesome ingredients. The recipes and tips that follow emphasize the natural sweetness of fresh fruits and vegetables and *small amounts of natural sweeteners*. All of the following recipes avoid the denatured ingredients so common in popular American treats, and the goodness of the natural ingredients shines through in better taste and nutrition. It is my hope that these tips will stimulate your awareness and creativity to make desserts with life-giving foods full of nutrients.

We have all heard of desserts that are "to die for." This chapter will give you desserts to live for.

fabulous fruits

328. Plain fresh fruit is a dessert all by itself. What could be more delicious than a bowl of just-picked strawberries in the spring, a succulent piece of watermelon on a hot summer afternoon, or a crisp, juicy apple on an autumn day? Absolutely nothing, as far as I'm concerned. "Just fruit" is just perfect for satisfying your sweet tooth naturally.

329. Ripeness is the key for enjoying fruit to its utmost. We've all tasted the difference between a mealy, bitter grapefruit and a juicy one that needs no sugar at all because it's perfect just the way it is. There's just no sense in buying fruit before (or after) its time.

330. Get to know what's in season. The availability and ripeness of fruits will vary from region to region, but the following chart gives some indication of when to buy produce at its prime. If you're ever in doubt, don't be afraid to ask the produce manager at your grocery store for his/her recommendations.

Apples:	September–December
Apricots:	June–August
Banana:	Year-round
Blackberries:	May–August
Blueberries:	May–September
Cherries:	June–August
Cranberries:	October–December
Grapefruit:	December–March
Grapes:	August–November
Mangoes:	May–September
Melons:	May–September
Oranges:	December–March
Papayas:	June–September
Peaches/Nectarines:	June–August
Pears:	November–February
Pineapple:	March–June
Plums:	May–October

Raspberries:	May–July
Strawberries:	April–July
Tangerines:	November–February
Watermelon:	May–August

331. Presentation is another key to enjoyment. When you arrange fruit in a colorful and appetizing way, not only does the fruit taste better, but the whole experience becomes a whole lot "sweeter."

332. Fresh fruit is tops in the taste department and frozen fruit is second best. Canned fruit is a distant third. I recommend limiting the use of canned fruit, but if you buy it for convenience, be sure to buy it packed in its own juices or, better yet, in water. Canned fruit in heavy syrup has almost twice the sugar of the juice-packed variety.

333. If you accidentally buy a syrup-sweetened can of fruit, put the fruit in a strainer and rinse it well with filtered water. This will help send some of those extra sugars down the drain.

334. Instead of putting sugar on top of half a grapefruit, spread one teaspoon of olive oil over it. Then let it stand for several hours before serving. The oil will neutralize the acid in the grapefruit and increase its sweetness.

335. For a new twist to an old staple, serve honeydew melon with lime slices. Squeezing lime on it gives the melon a new, refreshing flavor.

336. **Rome Beauty, Golden Delicious, Jonathan, Pippin, and Winesap** are all good baking apples. To make a baked apple (or a baked pear), preheat the oven to 350 degrees, core the fruit, fill it with the desired filling, and place 2 to 3 table- spoons of water in the baking dish with the fruit. Cover, or baste fruit with liquid several times during baking, and bake for 45–55 minutes, or until fruit is tender when pierced with a fork. Tasty, sugar-free filling ingredients to add include chopped walnuts or pecans; grated lemon or orange zest; cinnamon, nutmeg, cloves, or allspice; vanilla extract; or mint extract for a refreshing change of pace. *One Sweet Tooth.* 🦷

337. **For a slightly sweeter filling, for your baked apples,** try adding 1 tablespoon unsweetened apple juice; 1 tea- spoon maple syrup and ½ teaspoon maple extract; 1 table- spoon raisins, currants, or chopped dates; 1 tablespoon date "sugar"; or 1 tablespoon plain low-fat yogurt combined with 1 teaspoon of honey, a few drops of vanilla, and a dash of cin- namon. *Two Sweet Teeth.* 🦷 🦷

338. **When your taste buds want something new,** treat yourself to a fruit you haven't tried before. Boysenberries, guava, kiwi, and starfruit are exotic ways to break up your routine.

339. **Fruits vary in portion size because of their water and sugar contents.** Fruits with a lot of water (such as strawberries and watermelon) have a larger serving size (and also rank lower on the Glycemic Index) than fruits with less water such as bananas and dried fruits. As wonderful

and vitamin-packed as fruit is, don't go overboard eating it. Remember that fruit is still a source of sugars even though it's a natural one. Limit yourself to no more than two to three of the following portions of fruit per day:

Apple:	1 small
Apricots (fresh):	2 medium
Apricots (dried):	4 halves
Banana:	½ small
Berries (boysenberries, blackberries, blueberries, raspberries):	½ cup
Cantaloupe:	¼ (6-inch diameter)
Cherries:	10 large
Dates:	2
Figs (fresh):	1 large
Figs (dried):	1 small
Fruit cocktail (canned in juice):	½ cup
Grapefruit:	½ small
Honeydew melon:	⅛ (7-inch diameter)
Kiwi:	1 medium
Mango:	½ small
Nectarine:	1 small
Orange:	1 small
Papaya:	¾ cup
Peach:	1 medium
Pear:	1 small
Pineapple:	½ cup
Plums:	2 medium

Prunes:	2 medium
Raisins:	2 tablespoons
Strawberries:	¾ cup
Tangerine:	1 large
Watermelon:	1 cup

340. **An easy way to estimate the amount of fruit you're consuming** is to use your fist as a guide. The size of your fist equals about one cup of chopped fruit or one medium whole fruit.

fruit toppings

341. **Spreading unsweetened nut butter on apple, pear, or banana slices** is a way to enjoy these fruits but lessen their glycemic effects. This snack is a satisfying treat for anyone, but it is especially appreciated by diabetics and hypoglycemics. *One Sweet Tooth.* 🦷

342. **Toasted ground or slivered nuts or seeds** can also add a nice sugar-free finish to a bowl of fresh fruit. *One Sweet Tooth.* 🦷

343. **A few dashes of flavoring extract** can give fruit a dramatically new flavor, as you'll see in this easy, time-tested recipe from *Beyond Pritikin. One Sweet Tooth.* 🦷

VANILLA PEARS 𝕎

4 pears, cored, peeled, and halved
1 tablespoon water
1 teaspoon ground allspice
1 teaspoon vanilla extract

Preheat oven to 325 degrees. Place pears and water in baking dish. Sprinkle with allspice and drizzle each pear half with ⅛ teaspoon vanilla extract. Cover and bake about 20 minutes. *Serves 4.* 𝕎
Variation: Fresh peaches, plums, or nectarines can be used when in season.

344. **The healthiest topping I know of** is unsweetened low-fat yogurt with a pinch of Flora-Key added to slightly sweeten it. (See tip 71 for more information about FOS-containing Flora-Key.) Try this the next time you want something slightly sweet on fresh fruit. This topping is beneficial for almost everyone, but especially for individuals afflicted with yeast or parasitic infections or any type of digestive upset. The Flora-Key with the yogurt supplies friendly bacteria for the digestive tract, and the FOS feed the beneficial bacteria and help them multiply and thrive. *One Sweet Tooth.* 𝕎

345. **Other yogurt topping ideas** include mixing plain yogurt with ½ teaspoon vanilla extract and a dash or two of cinnamon, or with ¼ teaspoon almond extract and toasted chopped almonds, or with ¾ teaspoon coconut extract and 1 tablespoon unsweetened coconut. *One Sweet Tooth.* 𝕎

346. **Creamy frosting,** such as the frostings in either tip 377 or 378, makes a delicious dip for fresh strawberries. *Two Sweet Teeth.* 🦷🦷

347. **Serve your fruit Hawaiian style:** Top it with a tablespoon of unsweetened coconut milk. *One Sweet Tooth.* 🦷

348. **Or do as British royalty do:** Serve berries with fresh cream. *One Sweet Tooth.* 🦷

349. **For special occasions,** serve fruit with whipped cream made with a teaspoon or two of honey instead of confectioners' sugar. *Two Sweet Teeth.* 🦷🦷

350. **Pureed fresh fruit,** either by itself or combined with yogurt, makes a colorful and dressy topping for a fruit salad. In this recipe, Harriet Roth, author of *Deliciously Low,* shows us how to make an elegant dessert for a dinner party of fifteen without any fuss. *Two Sweet Teeth.* 🦷🦷

LAST-MINUTE FRUIT MÉLANGE 🦷🦷

1 pint fresh strawberries, washed and hulled
1 tablespoon unsweetened apple juice concentrate
¼ cup plain yogurt
1 teaspoon vanilla extract
1 20-ounce package frozen unsweetened peach slices
1 20-ounce package frozen unsweetened blueberries
1 20-ounce package frozen unsweetened Bing cherries

2 bananas, peeled and sliced (optional)
Fresh mint sprigs

To make strawberry-yogurt dressing, place strawberries, juice concentrate, yogurt, and vanilla in blender or food processor. Process until pureed. Place in covered container in refrigerator until serving time. About 30 minutes before serving time, place frozen peaches, blueberries, and cherries in an attractive glass serving bowl. When ready to serve, add dressing to fruit and mix gently. Sliced bananas may be added at this time if desired. Garnish with sprigs of fresh mint and serve in glass coupes or small Chinese lotus bowls. *Serves 15.* 🦷 🦷

---

veg out for dessert

351. **Sweet, starchy vegetables** are ideal ingredients for making desserts without concentrated sweeteners. Such vegetables as sweet potatoes, winter squash, pumpkin, carrots, parsnips, Jerusalem artichokes, and beets all provide subtle sweetness chock-full of nutrients and fiber and can be used to make everything from substantial sweet breads to whipped mousse desserts.

352. **Use mashed spaghetti squash** as a base for pudding. This tip comes from Barbara Anderson, one of my ardent Fat Flushers. The beauty of this dish lies in the endless variations that can be created by trying various fruits. *One Sweet Tooth.* 🦷

FAMOUS SPAGHETTI SQUASH PUDDING WITH MIXED BERRY PUREE 🦷

2 eggs
1 scoop vanilla Fat Flush Whey Protein
2 teaspoons ground cinnamon
2 packets stevia powder plus extra for puree if desired
3 cups cooked spaghetti squash
1 cup frozen mixed berries

Mix eggs in blender on low speed. Add whey, cinnamon, and 2 packets stevia powder and blend well on low speed. Add spaghetti squash and blend on high speed until well combined. Lightly coat a glass pie pan with olive oil spray. Sprinkle ½ cup frozen berries into pan. Pour spaghetti squash mixture into pan. Bake at 350 degrees for 20–30 minutes, or until well set. To make the puree, heat or defrost ½ cup frozen berries until softened. Puree to desired consistency. Sweeten with stevia powder if desired. Serve pudding hot or cold with berry puree. *Makes 2 servings.* 🦷

353. **Or serve baked winter squash with hot cinnamon syrup** for another delicious vegetable-based dessert. To make enough syrup for four servings, heat together 5 tablespoons of barley malt or rice syrup, 1 to 2 tablespoons butter, and a generous dash of cinnamon in a saucepan. Serve the squash with toasted nuts of your choice and pour the syrup on top. Remember, the butter and nuts in this dessert are good to include because their fat content helps slow down the body's response to the sweet syrup. *Two Sweet Teeth.* 🦷 🦷

354. **If you have a juicer gathering dust,** brush it off and start making vegetable juices again—to use in recipes. Experiment with using fresh carrot juice or carrot-beet juice in place of fruit juice concentrates in recipes. This cuts the sugar and gives you a healthy dose of beta-carotene to boot.

355. **Here's an idea for a frozen parsnip dessert** that came from my mentor, Dr. Hazel Parcells, when she was in her mid-eighties. *One Sweet Tooth.* 🦷

FROZEN PARSNIP DESSERT 🦷

2 cups cubed parsnip
1 pint heavy whipping cream
2 teaspoons honey
½ teaspoon vanilla extract
¼ teaspoon ground cardamom
Toasted walnut pieces

Thoroughly clean parsnips and freeze them in the freezer. When the parsnips are frozen, grate them or put them through a ricer so they have the consistency of shredded coconut. Whip the whipping cream very stiff and add the honey, vanilla, and cardamom. Fold the grated parsnips into the whipped cream, pour into 4 individual serving glasses, top with toasted walnut pieces, and chill. *Serves 4.* 🦷

tips for better baking

356. **When a recipe calls for 1 cup of sugar,** use more nutritious Sucanat in equal amounts or, better yet, reduce the amount of Sucanat by one-third to one-half of the sugar called for in the recipe and use other ingredients as the recipe suggests.

357. **You also can use date "sugar"** instead of sugar in the same way.

358. **For a less sweet version of one of your favorite recipes,** use brown rice syrup powder in equal proportions to the amount of sugar indicated.

359. **Fructose is sweeter than sugar;** ⅓ to ⅔ cup fructose will give the same sweetening power as 1 cup of sugar. Use fructose primarily in chilled and frozen desserts. It tastes sweeter in cold dishes than in hot ones.

360. **To use liquid sweeteners in a recipe that calls for sugar,** substitute ½ to ¾ cup honey, maple syrup, molasses, or fruit juice concentrate for 1 cup of sugar and decrease the other liquids in the recipe by ¼ cup for each ¾ cup of sweetener.

> **✻ *Bonus Tip*** If your honey ever crystallizes, simply set the jar in a bowl of hot water and the crystals will dissolve.

361. **You can also use 1½ cups of barley malt or rice syrup** in place of 1 cup of sugar and reduce the liquid in a recipe by 1 to 2 tablespoons.

---

* ***Bonus Tip*** To help sticky sweeteners such as barley malt or honey slip out of measuring spoons or cups, lightly oil your utensils or spray them with nonstick cooking spray before using.

---

362. **To use stevia in recipes,** use ½ to 1 teaspoon in place of 1 cup of sugar and add 1 to 2 tablespoons extra liquid. (For more about stevia, see tip 70.) Because of the strong after-taste of most stevia powders, you may wish to use stevia only in recipes that contain strongly flavored ingredients like carob. Stevia-sweetened baked goods don't brown, so be aware that you will need to time your baking a little more carefully and check for doneness by touch.

363. **To cut down the amount of honey, maple syrup, molasses, or juice concentrate** in a recipe, reduce the amount of sweetener by half and substitute unsweetened applesauce or mashed sweet potato for the other half.

364. **Slash the sugar even further** by using all unsweetened applesauce, pureed fruit, or pureed sweet potatoes.

365. **Reduce it further still** by mixing half unsweetened apple-sauce or pureed fruit with half water or herbal tea. Stevia tea works well in these kinds of cases where the least amount of sweetening is desired.

366. **Rice milk, soy milk, almond milk, or amasake** are four other ingredients that can lend their subtle, creamy sweetness to recipes when you want to eliminate more concentrated sweeteners.

367. **Know the sugar content of the sweeteners you're considering using.** The following list gives you the grams of sugars in 1 tablespoon of each sweetener, rounded to the nearest half gram. Since brands sometimes vary in sugar content, some sweeteners have a range of grams of sugars listed.

    Honey: 16–18 grams (17 grams on average)
    Fructose: 12–15 grams
    Blackstrap molasses: 11–15 grams
    Maple syrup: 13 grams
    Liquid FruitSource: 11 grams
    Granular FruitSource: 7.5 grams
    Apple juice concentrate: 7.5 grams
    Other juice concentrates: 5.5–8.5 grams
    All-fruit spread: 1–12 grams (9 grams average)
    Unsweetened apple butter: 4–8 grams
    Barley malt: 6 grams
    Brown rice syrup: 5 grams
    Rice syrup powder: 4 grams
    Sucanat: 3 grams

Date "sugar": 3 grams
Amazake brand amasake: 2 grams
Unsweetened apple juice: 2 grams
Other juices: 1.5–2 grams
Unsweetened applesauce: 1.5 grams
Other fruit-flavored applesauces: 1.5 grams
Rice milk, soy milk, and almond milk: 0.5–1 gram

368. **Use rosewater or orange blossom water** in place of vanilla or in place of 1 teaspoon of sweetener to delicately flavor cakes and cookies.

369. **Don't just replace white sugar in a recipe;** replace white flour as well. For every cup of white flour called for, use ⅞ cup whole-wheat flour or whole-wheat pastry flour.

370. **Experiment with other nutritious whole-grain flours,** which can add new flavor and texture to your baked goods. For variety, try one of the following substitutions in place of one cup of whole-wheat flour:

1 cup multigrain flour
1⅓ cups ground rolled oats
⅝ cup brown rice flour plus ½ cup rye flour
½ cup potato flour plus ½ cup rye flour
1¼ cups rye flour
¾ cup brown rice flour plus ⅓ cup amaranth flour
1 cup kamut flour
1 cup spelt flour

371. **Try substituting chestnut flour** in cake and cookie recipes in place of part of whatever flour you're using.

Chestnut flour is a wholesome way of adding extra lightness, creaminess, and sweetness to baked goods.

have your cake

372. Dinner quick breads can double nicely as subtly sweet desserts. My hypoallergenic Spelt Soda Bread succeeds in both roles. If you would like to dress it up for a sweeter dessert, serve it with Whipped Cream Frosting or Pineapple Frosting in tip 378 or 380. *Two Sweet Teeth.* 🦷🦷

SPELT SODA BREAD 🦷🦷

2 cups spelt flour

¼ teaspoon baking soda

½ teaspoon salt

6 tablespoons chilled butter

1 cup raisins

¼ cup chopped walnuts

½ to ⅓ cup almond milk

1 ounce soft tofu

1 tablespoon honey

¼ to ½ cup garbanzo flour (for kneading)

Olive oil spray

Preheat oven to 350 degrees. Mix together flour, baking soda, and salt. Cut in the chilled butter; stir in the raisins and walnuts. In a small bowl, blend the almond milk with the tofu and honey. Mix together the wet and dry ingredients. Knead briefly, adding in the garbanzo flour a little at a time as necessary to make the dough smooth and elastic. Shape the dough into a round loaf and place on a baking sheet that has been lightly coated with olive oil. Cut a large cross in the top of the loaf; spray lightly with olive oil. Bake for 50 minutes. Serve warm. *Serves 4.* 🦷🦷

373. **Whole-grain Belgian waffles for dessert?** You bet. They can substitute as easy fill-ins for shortcake when berries are in season and the idea of strawberry shortcake is beckoning. Van's makes a good line of frozen waffles you can heat up and use for such a purpose. Van's waffles contain no preservatives or cholesterol. Their latest creation, Hearty Oats waffles, contain the antioxidant power of one pomegranate, 4 grams of protein and fiber, and 1000 mg omega-3s, and are a good source of calcium. They also make a Carb Manager Waffle, Gourmet Waffle, Belgain Waffle, Organic Waffle (Blueberry and Soy Flax), Wheat Free Waffle, and Mini Waffles. Visit www.vanswaffles.com.

374. **What's carrot cake without the concentrated sweetening** of sugar, honey, or juice concentrate? Still very good when both moistness and varying textures are components of the cake. In this recipe from *Hot Times,* I use date "sugar," honey, and pureed fruits to give bursts of natural sweetness in every bite. *Two Sweet Teeth.* 🦷🦷

CARROT CAKE FOR A CROWD 🦷🦷

3 large carrots
1 large egg
⅜ cup oil
1 8-ounce can crushed pineapple in its own juice
1 cup raisins
1 teaspoon vanilla extract
1½ cups whole-wheat flour
1 teaspoon ground cinnamon
¼ teaspoon ground nutmeg
¼ teaspoon ground allspice
½ teaspoon salt
1½ teaspoons baking powder

Scrub and grate the carrots. Measure 1 cup and set aside. Spray an 8-inch-square baking pan with cooking spray. In a blender, combine egg, oil, pineapple and juice, raisins, and vanilla. Process until raisins are finely chopped. Measure flour, spices, salt, and baking powder into a large mixing bowl. Stir well. Add blended mixture and grated carrots to dry ingredients, mixing until batter is uniform. Spread batter into pan and bake at 350 degrees for 45–50 minutes or until cake tester comes out clean. Cool. Refrigerate. *Serves 8 to 10 people.* 🦷🦷

375. Want to treat yourself to a rich piece of cake but don't have time to bake? That's when individual thaw-and-serve portions of Amy's Cakes come in handy. Wholesome ingredients and no-fuss preparation—now that's my idea of pure indulgence! *Three Sweet Teeth.* 🦷🦷🦷

376. Decadent chocolate desserts are possible without refined sugar. This delicious recipe, courtesy of the Chatfield's company, will satisfy even the most confirmed chocolate lovers. *Three Sweet Teeth.* 🦷 🦷 🦷

CATHERINE'S FAVORITE
CHOCOLATE CAKE 🦷 🦷 🦷

1⅔ cups whole-wheat flour

¾ cup date "sugar"

¼ cup unsweetened cocoa powder

1 teaspoon baking soda

½ teaspoon salt

1 cup water

⅓ cup oil

1 teaspoon vinegar

1 teaspoon vanilla extract

Heat oven to 350 degrees. Mix flour, date "sugar," cocoa powder, baking soda, and salt with a fork in an ungreased 8-inch baking dish. Mix in remaining ingredients. Bake until a wooden toothpick inserted in the center comes out clean, about 35–40 minutes. *Serves 8 to 10 people.* 🦷 🦷 🦷

Note: You can also use Sucanat in place of date "sugar" in this recipe.

icing on the cake

377. A frosting suitable even for most sugar-restricted diets is Yogurt Cheese Icing, suggested by Janet Warrington in her book *Sweet and Natural*. To make the icing, combine enough pureed fruit with Yogurt Cheese (from tip 106) to make a mixture that you can spread thinly over cake. *One Sweet Tooth.* 🦷

378. Whipped cream used as a frosting is dressy despite being simple. Whether sweetened with honey, maple syrup, mashed banana, pureed fruit, or stevia powder—or even when it is used unsweetened—whipped cream works well on a wide variety of cakes. *One to Two Sweet Teeth.* 🦷–🦷 🦷

379. There is up to a cup of sugar in the typical cream cheese–based icing. Nancy Burrows, author of *Allergy Cooking Tricks and Treasures*, suggests making a low-sugar version of this popular favorite by softening an 8-ounce package of cream cheese in a mixer with one of the following: 1–2 teaspoons honey or maple syrup; 1–2 tablespoons orange juice; 1–2 teaspoons honey and 1 tablespoon fresh lemon juice; or 1 teaspoon vanilla extract and 1 teaspoon sweetener. If the mixture is too thick to spread easily, add a few tablespoons of water or milk to create the consistency you want. *One to Two Sweet Teeth.* 🦷–🦷 🦷

380. Here's a slightly sweeter version of cream cheese frosting that will compliment the Carrot Cake for a Crowd in tip 374. *One Sweet Tooth.* 🦷

PINEAPPLE FROSTING 🦷

3 ounces cream cheese, softened
1 8-ounce can crushed pineapple in its own juice,
drained, with juice reserved
¼ packet Stevia Plus

In a medium bowl, beat together the cream cheese, 2 tablespoons of the reserved pineapple juice, and stevia. Fold in crushed pineapple and refrigerate until it's thick enough to spread. *Makes 1 cup.* 🦷

381. **Kozlowski Farms apple butter or fruit spread** can also be used as an instant way to frost cakes.

382. **Or create a quick nut-butter cake glaze.** Just add a little maple syrup or honey, vanilla extract, and/or carob powder to the nut butter, mix together, and spread.

383. **When a special occasion calls for a splurge,** try this versatile, easy-to-make frosting that's rich in flavor but still lower in sugars than most traditional frostings. It comes from *Kid Smart: Raising a Healthy Child* by Cheryl Townsley. *Three Sweet Teeth.* 🦷🦷🦷

CAROB OR CHOCOLATE FROSTING 🦷🦷🦷

½ cup milk, almond milk, soy milk, or rice milk
¼ cup unsweetened carob or cocoa powder

2 tablespoons almond butter

3 to 4 tablespoons maple syrup

4 teaspoons arrowroot powder, or more as needed

¼ cup milk, almond milk, soy milk, or rice milk

Combine ¼ cup milk, carob or cocoa, almond butter, and maple syrup in a blender and blend until smooth. Transfer to a small pan. Stir in arrowroot and remaining ¼ cup milk. Heat on low, stirring occasionally, until the mixture thickens to almost a frosting consistency (about 5 to 7 minutes), then remove from heat. It will thicken a little more as it cools. *Makes enough for one 9-inch-square cake.* 🦷 🦷 🦷

384. **Instead of frosting a cake,** lightly dust one with coconut "sugar" (unsweetened shredded coconut finely ground in a blender).

385. **Or use powdered vanilla sugar,** a tasty topping you can make from recycled vanilla beans. After you've used vanilla beans, wipe them with a towel and allow them to dry on a plate overnight. Scrape away the little clumps of seeds from the pods and rub the clumps between your fingers to break them up. Add the seeds and plunge the pods into a jar of any dry sweetener—such as date "sugar," rice syrup powder, or Sucanat—and allow the vanilla flavor and aroma to penetrate the sugar for four to five days. You can sprinkle vanilla sugar on top of cream cheese as a cake topping or, for special occasions, powder it in a blender to lightly dust cakes.

386. **If you think frosting is the only way you can decorate cakes,** think again. Scraped carrot twirls, nuts, or

sliced fruit artfully arranged on top of cakes make delightfully attractive, low-sugar presentations. Other especially impressive decorations are pesticide-free edible flowers such as brightly colored pansies, rose petals, marigolds, or nasturtiums.

pies and crisps

387. There's no nicer way of enjoying the fruit in season than making a fresh fruit pie. Unfortunately, most fruit pies are filled with as much as 1½ cups sweetener in addition to all that delicious fruit. This recipe from Carol Nostrand's *Junk Food to Real Food* avoids all that added sugar, but you'll never miss it. Simply by soaking fresh apples and raisins in lemon juice and cinnamon, she has created an apple pie filling that ranks right up there with the best of them. *Two Sweet Teeth.* 🦷 🦷

RAW FRUIT PIE WITH
APPLE FILLING 🦷 🦷

2 cups ground walnuts
¾ pound soft dried dates, pitted and chopped
3 large Golden Delicious apples, peeled, cored, quartered,
and sliced into ¼-inch-thick segments
¾ cup raisins
Juice of 1½ small lemons (about 4 tablespoons)
1 teaspoon ground cinnamon

To make the crust, blend walnuts to a fine powder in a food processor or blender. Chop the dates in a food processor or blender. Then knead the crust ingredients together. Press into a 10-inch pie plate. Refrigerate overnight to help the crust harden. Also overnight, soak the apples and raisins in the lemon juice and cinnamon. The next day spoon the filling into the pie crust and serve. *Makes one 10-inch pie.* 🦷 🦷

388. **When converting your favorite pie recipes** using the tips in this book, start with the crust. Remember, refined white flour is out; whole grains are in. Here's a basic Whole-Wheat Crust that you can use in all your favorite recipes. It comes from *Sweet and Natural* by Janet Warrington.

WHOLE-WHEAT CRUST

1 cup whole-wheat flour
¼ teaspoon salt
¼ teaspoon oil
2 tablespoons ice water

In a medium bowl, stir flour and salt with a fork to thoroughly mix. Combine oil and water in a measuring cup and pour it into the flour mixture. Stir until all ingredients are moistened. Pour the pastry mixture into a pie plate and flatten it across the bottom and up the sides of the plate using your fingers, the back of a spoon, or the outside of an empty measuring cup. Be careful to distribute the pastry evenly. For an empty shell, bake at 400 degrees for 15 minutes. *Makes enough for 1 pie.*

389. **If you're in a hurry,** give yourself the luxury of using a wholesome frozen whole-wheat crust. Mother Nature's Goodies makes a good one you should be able to find in your local health-food store.

390. **Heat-and-serve frozen pies** are also available from Mother Nature's Goodies. They're a good alternative to most other store-bought pies, but still quite sweet. *Three Sweet Teeth.* 🦷 🦷 🦷

391. **Using a combination of fruit-flavored applesauce and fruit spread** as sweeteners produces flavorful desserts that are much lower in sugars than the same desserts sweetened with sugar, honey, or juice concentrate. This recipe is not quite a cobbler, but it is not your typical pie recipe either because it's much simpler. Mixing everything together instead of making a separate pie crust and pie filling saves time and effort. That's why it's "magic." *Two Sweet Teeth.* 🦷 🦷

MAGIC PEACH COBBLER PIE 🦷 🦷

1 cup brown rice flour

¼ to ½ teaspoon salt

¼ teaspoon ground nutmeg

1 teaspoon ground cinnamon

1 teaspoon cream of tartar

⅓ cup oil

½ cup peach applesauce

3 tablespoons peach fruit spread
1 teaspoon almond extract
1 teaspoon baking soda
2 tablespoons boiling water
4 cups fresh peaches, peeled and thinly sliced

Oil and lightly dust with flour a 10-inch pie pan. Stir together the dry ingredients in a large bowl. Then preheat the oven to 350 degrees. Combine the oil, peach applesauce, fruit spread, and almond extract, then add them to the flour mixture and mix well. Combine the baking soda and boiling water, stir to dissolve, and add to the batter. Quickly fold in the peaches, then scrape the batter into the pie pan and place in oven. Bake 40–50 minutes, or until pie is brown and peaches are tender. *Serves 8 to 10 people.* 🦷🦷

392. A small serving of a fresh dessert is sometimes all you or your guests want. Here's a recipe for an Apple, Cranberry, and Pear Crisp that's especially nice for entertaining. *Two Sweet Teeth.* 🦷🦷

APPLE, CRANBERRY, AND PEAR CRISP 🦷🦷

2 baking apples, peeled, cored, and sliced
(Granny Smith, Gala, etc.)
2 pears, peeled, cored, and sliced
½ cup fresh or frozen cranberries
⅓ cup plus 1 tablespoon oat flour

2 teaspoons Stevia Plus
2 tablespoons fresh lemon juice
1 scoop vanilla Fat Flush Whey Protein
½ to 1 teaspoon cinnamon
2 tablespoons butter, chilled
½ cup steel-cut oats, soaked in ½ cup hot water until softened
¼ cup chopped walnuts

Preheat the oven to 375 degrees. Coat an 8-by-8-inch baking dish with cooking spray. In a medium bowl, mix the apples, pears, and cranberries. In a small bowl, combine 1 tablespoon oat flour and ½ teaspoon Stevia Plus. Stir in the lemon juice, mixing until the stevia is dissolved. Pour over the fruit and toss until well coated. Set the filling aside.

Make the crust. In a separate bowl, combine ⅓ cup oat flour, whey protein, 1½ teaspoons Stevia plus, and the cinnamon. Cut in the butter, using a pastry blender or 2 knives, until only small lumps remain. Stir in the soaked oats, draining any remaining water. The oat flour mixture should resemble thick paste; stir in a small amount of additional water if needed. Fold in the walnuts.

Pour the fruit mixture into the prepared pan and spread the crust mixture over the top. Bake 45 minutes, or until brown and crispy on top. For a pretty finish, place under the broiler for 1 minute, watching carefully. Let cool for 10 minutes before serving. *Makes 8 servings.* 🦷 🦷

393. Avoid store-bought cheesecake: The main ingredient is cheap, refined sugar. The following recipe for cheesecake is simple and requires no baking. *Two Sweet Teeth.* 🦷 🦷

BANANA CHEESECAKE IN A CUP 🦷🦷

1 cup large-curd cottage cheese
2 ripe bananas, frozen
¼ teaspoon vanilla extract
1 tablespoon honey
4 teaspoons chopped toasted pecans
Cinnamon

Puree the cottage cheese in a blender or food processor until smooth. Add the frozen bananas, vanilla, and honey, processing just until the bananas are incorporated. Divide into small bowls. Sprinkle with chopped pecans and cinnamon; serve immediately. *Serves 4.* 🦷🦷

satisfying cookies

394. When I want to treat myself to a cookie, the last thing I want is the fat-free kind—for two reasons. First, as a consumer who likes the taste of good food, I know I won't be satisfied with the fatless, sawdust-textured variety. Second, as a nutritionist who has studied the sugar issue for more than twenty years, I know that "fat-free" almost always means "more sugar than you bargained for." The key to healthy cookie enjoyment, I have found, is to treat yourself to one with *moderate* amounts of both sugar and fat—and hopefully some fiber as well.

395. Chocolate chip is the cookie of choice for most Americans when they want a treat. It's clear Americans are crazy about chocolate chips: approximately 70 percent of the population actually keeps a package of semisweet chocolate morsels at home to bake with. The sugar-smart way to still enjoy chocolate chip cookies but get the sugar out of them is to use malt-sweetened chips such as those made by Sunspire or Chatfield's instead of the sugar-sweetened ones made by Nestlé or Hershey's.

396. Adding high-fiber ingredients such as oats to cookie recipes is a good way to slow down the body's response to the sugar in these sweets. This recipe from nutritionist Melissa Diane Smith, for moist, scrumptious Oatmeal Chocolate Chip Cookies, illustrates this concept well. *Two Sweet Teeth.* 🦷🦷

OATMEAL CHOCOLATE
CHIP COOKIES 🦷🦷

1 cup raisins (golden raisins produce a lighter-color cookie)
1 cup unsweetened apple juice
¼ cup oil
1 cup oat flour *or* finely ground oats
1 cup oats
½ teaspoon baking soda
¾ teaspoon ground cinnamon
¾ cup malt-sweetened chocolate chips or carob chips
½ cup chopped walnuts (optional)

Soak the raisins in the juice overnight. The next day, puree them together in a blender, then add the oil and blend again briefly. Combine the rest of the ingredients in a bowl and mix thoroughly. Add the raisin-juice mixture and stir just until combined. Drop heaping teaspoonfuls of the batter onto an ungreased baking sheet and bake at 375 degrees for 15–18 minutes, or until the cookies are lightly browned. *Makes about 36 cookies.* 🦷🦷

397. **If you want to avoid the blood-sugar-raising caffeine in chocolate chips,** substitute malt-sweetened carob chips for chocolate chips in the above recipe. *Two Sweet Teeth.* 🦷🦷

398. **If you're a macaroon fan,** try these cookies, which combine the subtle sweetening power of brown rice syrup powder, lemon extract, and grated lemon peel to produce delightfully light Lemony Almond Macaroon Drops. *One Sweet Tooth.* 🦷

LEMONY ALMOND
MACAROON DROPS 🦷

1 cup ground blanched almonds
3 egg whites
1 tablespoon lemon extract or vanilla extract
4½ tablespoons brown rice syrup powder
1 tablespoon grated lemon peel
21 whole almonds

Mix together the ground blanched almonds, egg whites, flavoring extract, brown rice syrup powder, and lemon peel. Mix until well blended, then chill the dough for one hour. Drop by heaping teaspoons onto an oiled cookie sheet. Press a whole almond into the top of each cookie and bake at 350 degrees until light brown, about 5 minutes. Cookies will harden more as they cool. *Makes 21 cookies.* 🦷

399. Naturally sweetened packaged cookies that taste like homemade are available, and one of the best brands is a line called Pamela's. With varieties ranging from ginger cookies to butter shortbread to almond anise biscotti, Pamela's cookies are so wholesome that usually one cookie is all you need for total satisfaction. They're available in natural food stores nationwide. *Two Sweet Teeth.* 🦷 🦷

400. The sweetening power of plain mashed banana continues to amaze me. Mashed banana is the only sweetener in these tried-and-true cookies, which are one of my staff members' favorites. *Two Sweet Teeth.* 🦷 🦷

CHEWY BANANA-OAT COOKIES 🦷 🦷

1½ cups oats
½ cup whole-wheat pastry flour, oat flour, or millet flour
½ teaspoon salt
¼ teaspoon baking soda
Pinch ground cinnamon (optional)

2 tablespoons chopped nuts or raisins

2 medium bananas, mashed (about 1 cup)

⅜ cup oil (¼ cup plus 2 tablespoons oil)

Preheat oven to 350 degrees. Mix dry ingredients. In a separate bowl, mix mashed bananas and oil, then add to the dry ingredients. Drop by heaping teaspoons onto an unoiled cookie sheet. Bake 10–15 minutes. *Makes about 24 cookies.* 🦷 🦷

Note: These cookies freeze well. You can double this recipe and freeze some for future treats.

401. **To make Oatmeal Harvest Cookies,** use 1 cup of mashed sweet potato or mashed acorn squash in place of the mashed banana. *One Sweet Tooth.* 🦷

> **✱ *Bonus Tip*** You can also create other varieties of these whole-grain cookies by eliminating the oats and using rolled wheat flakes, barley flakes, rye flakes, spelt flakes, or kamut flakes instead.

natural candy

402. **Candy is a multibillion-dollar business** and one of the top three snack foods Americans consume. It's important to remember that candy gives us lots of calories but little

nutrition, yet manufacturers develop elaborate advertising campaigns and sponsorships to hook kids into the candy habit while they're still young and impressionable. Do your kids and yourself a favor by saying no to the heavily advertised, nutrient-poor commercial candies, and learn to satisfy your need for something sweet with the natural alternatives suggested in this section.

403. Great substitutes for hard candy are frozen grapes, raspberries, and blueberries. *One Sweet Tooth.* 🦷

404. So are dried fruits, which are nature's concentrated sources of natural sugars as well as vitamins, minerals, and fiber. *Three Sweet Teeth.* 🦷 🦷 🦷

* **Bonus Tip** It's worth it to seek out unsulfured dried fruits for treats. Commercial dried fruits treated with sulfur dioxide can produce unpleasant symptoms such as nausea, headaches, and rashes, and sometimes even more serious, life-threatening allergic reactions.

405. When a bite of *rich* candy is what you want, stuffed dates can naturally fulfill your wishes. Just pit a few dates and fill them with unsweetened peanut butter, almond butter, or cashew butter. You'll be surprised at how rich and filling these easy-to-make creations are. *Two Sweet Teeth.* 🦷 🦷

406. Here's another convincing example of how fruit can be candy. *Two Sweet Teeth.* 🦷 🦷

FRUIT CANDY 🦷 🦷

½ cup sesame seeds or chopped nuts
½ cup finely chopped dried fruit
¼ teaspoon ground cinnamon or more to taste
1 cup unsweetened nut butter or seed butter
½ cup unsweetened shredded coconut

Lightly toast sesame seeds or chopped nuts in a 275-degree oven for a few minutes until they're fragrant and golden brown, being careful not to burn them. Stir the seeds or chopped nuts, chopped dried fruit, and cinnamon together in a bowl. Gradually add nut or seed butter, using just enough to form a soft dough. Roll dough into small ball or log shapes, then gently roll each of them in shredded coconut. Place on a cookie sheet or platter and refrigerate until serving. *Makes 24 to 36 pieces.* 🦷 🦷

407. Other ingredients to experiment with when making no-bake dried-fruit candies are other nut butters or tahini; powdered grain-based coffee substitutes; vanilla, orange, or almond extracts; and peppermint, spearmint, or wintergreen oils.

408. Carob powder and shredded coconut are naturals in candy concoctions because they're both naturally sweet.

This simple recipe is adapted from my *Eat Fat, Lose Weight Cookbook. One Sweet Tooth.* 🦷

PEANUT BUTTER BALLS 🦷

½ cup natural crunchy peanut butter
½ cup flaxseed oil
½ cup shredded coconut
⅛ cup carob powder

Thoroughly mix peanut butter and flaxseed oil in a bowl. Stir in the coconut and carob powder. If mixture isn't thick enough, add more coconut. Form into balls. Serve immediately or cover and chill for later use. *Makes 6 servings.* 🦷

409. **In the mood for chocolate?** That could be because chocolate supplies b-phenethylamine, the same chemical your brain produces when you're in love. Fortunately, a bite or two of chocolate is usually all that you need for a treat. A small piece provides that same luscious feel in your mouth that a large piece does, and a mini-splurge can be so satisfying that it can act as a natural deterrent against overindulging.

410. **If you're going to treat yourself to chocolate,** make sure you choose a naturally sweetened variety instead of the usual candy bar made with refined sugar. Try splitting a CHOCOperfection bar with a friend. CHOCOperfection bars offer 95 percent fewer calories than traditional choco-

> ✳ ***Bonus Tip*** Tamera's truffles offer a 100 percent organic truffle high in the natural mood enhancer found in chocolate. Visit www.tamerastruffles.com or call 541-273-2212. This unique treats also contain E3Live (*Aphanizomenon flos-aquae*), a blue-green algae that contains more than sixty-four nutrients that are 97 percent absorbed by the body. Certified organic and kosher. For more information contact Vision, 888-800-7070, or visit www.e3live.com.

late bars because they contain erythritol instead of sugar. These bars have no effect on insulin levels and are high in natural fiber, so they actually help to suppress the appetite—imagine a chocolate bar that helps you control your weight! Plus this bar is diabetic- (and tooth-) friendly. Call Low Carb Specialties, Inc., 800-332-1773.

gelatins and puddings

411. J-E-L-L-O is nutrient-void S-U-G-A-R no matter how you look at it. If you or your kids are fond of this common American dessert, make it the healthier way with unsweetened fruit juice. Just add 1 tablespoon unflavored gelatin to 2 cups of any kind of warm, unsweetened fruit juice. Stir until the gelatin dissolves, then pour the gelatin mixture into serving cups and chill until set. *Three Sweet Teeth.* 🦷 🦷 🦷

> ✱ **Bonus Tip** If you make gelatin fruit salad, do not add fresh pineapple, papaya, guava, kiwi, figs, or gingerroot to the gelatin. These foods contain enzymes that prevent the gelatin from setting.

412. **Another, healthier gelatin** can be made with agar-agar, a seaweed gelatin, in place of animal gelatin. Combine 2 cups unsweetened juice and 2 tablespoons agar-agar flakes in a saucepan and boil for 30 seconds. Cool for 20 minutes, then refrigerate until set. *Three Sweet Teeth.* 🦷 🦷 🦷

413. **Whipping up this pudding is a dream** because it's so ridiculously simple to make but it is amazingly sweet, rich, and creamy even though it's only sweetened with banana. It's another recipe from *Sweet and Natural* by Janet Warrington. *One Sweet Tooth.* 🦷

PEANUT BUTTER PUDDING 🦷

1 small ripe banana
½ cup plain nonfat yogurt
½ cup natural peanut butter
¼ teaspoon vanilla extract
Pinch salt (optional)

Combine all ingredients in a blender. Process first on low speed, then on high until smooth. Pour into 4 individual serving dishes and refrigerate. Serve cold. *Serves 4.* 🦷

414. **Here's another blended dessert** that is a good substitute for sugar-sweetened, fruit-flavored yogurt. It was developed especially for this book by Holly Sollars, a former demonstration chef at Canyon Ranch health resort. *Two Sweet Teeth.* 🦷

FRUITY TOFU DELIGHT 🦷🦷

One 10.5-ounce package of Mori-Nu extra-firm
silken tofu
1½ cups unsweetened frozen cherries or other frozen fruit
¼ cup Kozlowski Farms cherry spread or
other flavor all-fruit spread

Place tofu in a blender on medium until smooth and silky, stopping occasionally to scrape unblended tofu from the sides of the blender container. Add frozen fruit and process, then add fruit spread and blend until smooth. Serve immediately, or chill for several hours for a firmer consistency. *Makes 2 to 3 servings.* 🦷🦷

415. **Another quick pudding** can be made by blending about 1 pound of drained tofu, a 16-ounce can of drained pineapple, and honey and vanilla to taste. *Two Sweet Teeth.* 🦷🦷

416. **Tapioca pudding is terrific,** especially when you replace the sugar in your favorite recipe with date "sugar," brown rice syrup powder, rice syrup, barley malt, honey, or maple syrup. *Two Sweet Teeth.* 🦷🦷

417. Bread pudding is another recipe that's easy to adapt. Use a natural sweetener in place of sugar and be sure to use whole-grain bread cubes instead of white bread cubes. *Two Sweet Teeth.* 🦷🦷

418. Rice pudding is delicious made with short-grain brown rice instead of white rice. (I think it's better.) I also like it because it's an easy way to use up leftover brown rice you have in the refrigerator and because you can make it in a variety of ways—in the Crock-Pot, in a saucepan on the stovetop, or baked in the oven. This recipe, from *Smart Breakfasts* by Jane Kinderlehrer, is a way to bake Brown Rice Pudding in the oven. *Two Sweet Teeth.* 🦷🦷

BROWN RICE PUDDING 🦷🦷

2 eggs
2 cups milk (2% milk makes a creamier pudding
than nonfat does)
¼ cup honey or rice syrup
1 teaspoon vanilla extract
1½ cups cooked short-grain brown rice
½ cup raisins
Pinch grated nutmeg and/or ground cinnamon

Preheat oven to 350 degrees. In a food processor or mixing bowl, blend together the eggs, milk, sweetener, and vanilla. Stir in the brown rice and raisins. Spoon into a 1-quart casserole and dust with nutmeg and/or cinnamon. Bake for 1 to 1½ hours. Pudding is done when a knife inserted in the center comes out clean. Serve hot with milk or cream, or chill and serve plain. *Serves 8.* 🦷🦷

---

frozen treats

419. **The light, refreshing sweetness of frozen pureed fruit** comes through whether you make it into a sorbet or a fruit pop. To make sorbet for four people, place about 2 cups of pureed fruit combined with 1 teaspoon of honey or a pinch of fructose in a plastic container and freeze for 2 hours. Take out and stir well, then return to the freezer to freeze completely. Allow it to sit for 15 minutes at room temperature before serving. Any kind of fruit works in this recipe, but sorbet made out of cantaloupe, mango, grapefruit, or berries seems particularly refreshing to me on hot summer days. *Two Sweet Teeth.* 🦷🦷

420. **To make a frozen fruit pop out of pureed fruit,** Carol Nostrand, author of *Junk Food to Real Food,* suggests blending sliced fresh fruit (about 1½ fruit servings per person) with a little bit of water and pouring the fruit puree into ice-pop molds or leftover small juice concentrate cans. Put wooden sticks in the mold, then allow to freeze until solid. To serve, run warm water over the outside of the mold or can and the fruit pop will slip out. *Two Sweet Teeth.* 🦷🦷

421. Or make creamy fruit pops. Follow the instructions above except use 1 piece of fruit (for example, 1 chopped medium peach) blended with 3–4 tablespoons low-fat yogurt and ¼ teaspoon natural vanilla extract. *Two Sweet Teeth.* 🦷🦷

422. What tastes like frozen custard on the inside and nutty Swiss-almond ice cream on the outside? "Gone Nutty" Frozen Bananas—a perfect cool treat on a sticky summer afternoon. *Two Sweet Teeth.* 🦷🦷

"GONE NUTTY" FROZEN BANANAS 🦷🦷

¼ cup almond milk
3 tablespoons almond butter
¼ teaspoon almond extract
2 ripe bananas
½ cup lightly toasted ground almonds

Blend together the almond milk, almond butter, and almond extract in a blender. Peel the bananas, cut them in half, roll them in the almond milk mixture, then roll them in the almonds. Place on a small plate and freeze until solid. Allow to thaw for at least 15 minutes before eating. *Serves 4.* 🦷🦷

423. What's ice cream without refined sugar? Very good, and it's possible to make it even if you don't have an ice cream machine. In this tried-and-true recipe, Nancy Burrows, author of *Allergy Cooking Tricks and Treasures,* shows us how. *Three Sweet Teeth.* 🦷 🦷 🦷

VANILLA ICE CREAM 🦷 🦷 🦷

1 teaspoon gelatin
2 tablespoons cold water
1 12-ounce can unsweetened evaporated milk
⅓ cup honey or maple syrup
2 teaspoons vanilla extract

Sprinkle gelatin over cold water in a bowl. Let soften 10 minutes. Heat half of milk to very hot or scalding. (A double boiler prevents burning.) Add hot milk to gelatin mixture and stir to dissolve. Add remaining milk. Chill. (The freezer speeds up this step.) Whip cold mixture with electric mixer until soft peaks form, about 8–10 minutes. Add sweetener and vanilla and mix to incorporate thoroughly. Freeze in covered container. *Makes about 1³/₄ quarts.* 🦷 🦷 🦷

Variation: You can make mint ice cream by adding one drop of peppermint extract to the above recipe.

424. Chocolate ice cream without milk and sugar? Sure, it's easy when pureed bananas serve as a combination creamy base and sweetener. This delectable recipe comes from *The "I Can't Believe This Has No Sugar" Cookbook* by Deborah E. Buhr. *Three Sweet Teeth.* 🦷 🦷 🦷

CHOCOLATE ICE CREAM 🦷🦷🦷

4 bananas, peeled
4 ounces unsweetened chocolate
3 tablespoons water

In a bowl, mash the bananas. Melt chocolate with water in the top of a double boiler. Add melted chocolate and water to bananas, stir, and freeze before serving. *Serves 4.* 🦷🦷🦷

get the sugar out
when you eat out

*t*here is perhaps no greater challenge to reducing the sugar in your diet than getting the sugar out when you eat out. After all, when you decide to give yourself a break from cooking and let others cook for you instead, you give up some control in exchange for convenience (and perhaps also for ambience, sociability, and just plain pampering). You no longer choose every ingredient or how much of every ingredient is put into the food you are served. Hidden sugar can thus sneak into your food unless you develop the know-how to keep the sugar out.

A big part of keeping the sugar out when you eat out is knowing what to expect from the average eatery. For example, if you order pancakes at a typical restaurant, you should obviously not expect to be served whole-grain cakes and pure maple syrup. Similarly, if you order rice off a menu, it will be white rice; pasta off a menu will be white pasta; and bread off a menu will be white bread unless the menu specifically tells you otherwise. In addition, desserts will almost always be made with white flour and white sugar—the kinds we should all avoid—unless you go out of your way to get one at a natural food restaurant. The trick to avoiding these nutrient-poor carbohydrates when dining out, then, is either to frequent restaurants that offer whole-grain choices on the menu (something I try to do when I'm traveling) or to dine at other restaurants and just skip the processed starches as much as possible and emphasize more vegetables.

If you're like many people today, you may eat out more often than you eat in. Once you have an idea of what to expect when eating out, it is much easier to know what and how to order to avoid unwanted sugars. Knowing how to get low-sugar foods—whether at a fast-food chain, a Chinese restaurant, or a four-star gourmet restaurant—is a basic survival skill that all of us need to learn.

The tips in this chapter cover this important topic as well as the equally important subject of what foods you should take on short excursions and long trips. These tips will teach you how to eat nutritiously on the run so you can keep up a healthful pace.

getting what you want

425. **Don't be afraid to ask questions** such as "What's in that?" or "How is that prepared?" Remember that your waiter or waitress is at the restaurant to serve you. It's in the restaurant's best interests to have a satisfied customer, so don't feel sheepish about politely making special requests, particularly when your emotional and physical health depend upon it.

426. Pick and choose from the menu. If a food is on the menu, you should be able to get it, even though it may not be listed with the particular entrée you want. A grilled chicken breast, for example, may be topped with a sugar-rich barbecue sauce, while a pasta dish (made from white flour) might be teamed with a fresh tomato-and-basil sauce. You should be able to combine the best aspects of the two entrées and get a chicken breast topped with the tomato-basil sauce— an entrée that eliminates sugars and refined carbohydrates completely.

427. One of the toughest challenges when eating in restaurants today is avoiding processed carbohydrates such as white rice, pasta, and bread. It's easiest just to skip the starches and ask for a double order of veggies or salad instead.

428. Be clear about what you want and stress to your servers that you are following a diet in which you need to avoid sugar and other sweeteners. Restaurant servers are more likely to pay attention when you tell them that you *need* to avoid sugar instead of that you want to. (It should not matter whether you are eliminating sugar because of a yeast infection, heart disease, hypoglycemia, or just to feel your best. The restaurant should take your desire to avoid sugar as seriously as it does a diabetic's.)

429. Ask for a particularly accommodating server by name when making reservations at a restaurant you frequent. If you've gotten the kind of food and service you've wanted from that server before, you can expect to get it again. It's nice to have established a close enough relationship with your server to say, "I'll have the usual," and know that he or she will get your order right, no questions asked.

> ✳ ***Bonus Tip***   Be sure to reward your special server (or any accommodating server) with both praise and a generous tip. These will go a long way toward ensuring that you get the same quality service in the future.

430. Natural food restaurants are worth seeking out.
When you find one, you can be assured that the selections offered are made with fresh, wholesome ingredients. As a result, your meal is much less apt to contain hidden sugars. In addition, eating at a natural food restaurant often means you can treat yourself to tasty whole-grain dishes and naturally sweetened desserts that are simply not available at other restaurants.

menu savvy

431. Avoid the after-breakfast sugar blues by steering clear of these typical sugar-rich restaurant breakfast foods: pastries, croissants, and muffins; white toast, bagels, English muffins, and fruit jam; pancakes, waffles, and all of their accompaniments; fruit crêpes; granola and other sweetened cereals; fruit-flavored yogurt; and ham, bacon, and sausage.

432. **Don't be fooled into thinking "heart-healthy" symbols** on a restaurant menu necessarily mean "blood-sugar-healthy." In fact, as more and more restaurant chefs try to reduce the fat in the meals they prepare, they are increasingly using sugar-rich glazes, marinades, and sauces. A sugar-laden pineapple-teriyaki-glazed chicken breast may qualify for a little heart symbol on a menu, but it's not an entrée for balancing blood sugar levels. (We now know that it's not exactly heart-healthy either because too much sugar contributes to heart problems.)

433. **Watch out for key menu words and phrases** that signal too much sugar. Anytime a food is served with a sweet glaze or syrup, steer clear of it.

434. *Caramelized* is another term that usually means "sugarized."

435. **Avoid entrées that say they are served with the restaurant's "own special sweet sauce."** The main ingredient in many sweet sauces is usually refined sugar.

436. **The same is often true of barbecue sauces and honey-based mustards and salad dressings.** Pass up these disguised sugar sources whenever possible.

437. **Fruit sauces on entrées may sound healthy,** but they are apt to have a lot of empty-calorie sugar and wine in them and not much fruit. In general, ask that entrées be prepared without sugary sauces or at least ask for the sauce on the side.

438. **The safest salad dressing to order** as far as sugar is concerned is vinegar and oil or lemon wedges and oil. Creamy commercial dressings that restaurants buy in bulk are common sources of hidden sugars.

＊ *Bonus Tip* With the help of 2-ounce, watertight Tupperware containers known as Midgets, you can unobtrusively carry sugar-free dressings or unrefined oils with you just about anywhere you go.

439. **Limit ordering so-called light fare** such as pasta salad or fruit salad served with sherbet or frozen yogurt. Remember that these foods are light on nutrition and heavy on nutrient-poor sugars and processed carbohydrates.

440. **Don't forget that one glass of soda or juice** gives you more sugar than most of us should consume in a single day. Order instead bottled water, mineral water, soda water, or iced or hot teas.

441. **Avoid ordering desserts in restaurants,** where you can't control the amount and type of sweeteners put in them. If you don't want to seem antisocial, try inviting your dining companions to your house for a healthier dessert.

442. **Or order a bowl of berries or a fruit salad,** which are the safest choices at the restaurant. Even if you do not see fruit on the menu, don't hesitate to ask for it. Most good restaurants have fruit in the kitchen to use in other desserts or for garnishes. They usually are more than willing to serve it to you.

international insights

443. **Foreign cuisines not only offer variety** but also can offer healthy, low-sugar eating as long as you use sugar savvy when ordering. Not all ethnic food is low in sugar, but it is often more healthful and less processed than American fare, particularly dishes where lots of fresh vegetables are emphasized.

444. **If you decide to go Italian** (as I often do), try not to make refined pasta and refined bread the cornerstones of your meal. Choose instead deliciously prepared veal, chicken, fish, or shellfish with garlic and fresh herbs, and add a leafy green Italian salad and a medley of flavorful sautéed vegetables.

445. **When you want to eat Greek,** keep a few guidelines in mind. Avoid Greek pastries; limit your intake of white pasta, rice, and pita bread; and avoid dishes with honey-based sauces. Some good sugar-free Greek dishes to try include souvlaki, roast leg of lamb, chicken Athenian, shrimp Scorpios, and traditional Greek salad. Avgolemono (Greek egg-lemon soup) is particularly delicious and tastes sweet even though it contains no sugar.

446. **Chinese restaurants provide ample selections from which to choose** as long as you avoid sugar-containing sweet-and-sour, plum, and hoisin sauces. Request that no sugar be added to your meal during cooking. If your meal seems a little bland without any extra sugar, ask for hot mustard, minced garlic, scallions, or some Chinese five-spice powder from the kitchen to give your dish a little extra seasoning. Chinese five-spice powder is my particular favorite for sweetening a stir-fry without sugar.

447. **Japanese restaurants and Japanese steakhouses** can provide not only healthful food but also fun entertainment if they cook the food right at your table. When ordering, remember that any hibachi-style dish should be sugar-free, but not necessarily sukiyaki and teriyaki dishes. These are better avoided.

448. **When the restaurant you visit is French,** stay away from the French pastries and sweet dishes such as duck à

> * **Bonus Tip** Sushi is an increasingly popular offering at many Japanese restaurants. Although raw-fish-based sushi does not contain sugar, I do not recommend it because of the increasing amounts of parasites and contaminants found in seafood. To enjoy sushi from time to time, choose safe kinds made with avocado, cucumber, or cooked crab or shrimp.

l'orange. Especially healthy French selections include fish en papillote (fish cooked in its own juices with herbs), poached salmon, poulet aux fines herbes (roast chicken with herbs), bouillabaisse, ratatouille, and salad niçoise.

449. In the mood for Mexican food? Go ahead and enjoy it. Although some fast-food Mexican restaurants may add sugar to the food they serve, most good Mexican restaurants will not, so the main thing you have to avoid is tortillas made from refined flour. Opt for corn tortillas instead unless you're lucky enough to find a Mexican eatery or health food restaurant that uses whole-wheat tortillas. Good selections to order at Mexican restaurants include beef tostadas, chicken or beef fajitas, bean burritos, and taco salad.

450. Indian dishes sometimes contain small amounts of naturally occurring sweet foods such as raisins, but the amounts are usually small enough and balanced with enough protein and fat that they don't cause much of a blood sugar problem. Such dishes as chicken and lamb tandoori, korma, or curry can all fit nicely into a low-sugar way of life, and basmati rice–based biryanis or bean-based dals are good sources of healthful, unrefined complex carbohydrates.

on the run and on the road

451. **Limit your intake of typical fast food** because, although it may be fast, most of it is a disaster for anyone trying to avoid sugar, salt, and nonessential fat. French fries at fast-food outlets frequently are dipped in a sugar solution before frying, beef patties may have sugar added to them as a flavor enhancer, and breadings for fried chicken and fish usually are sugar-rich. Condiments such as ketchup, salad dressings, and "special sauces" aren't so special anymore when you realize that their key ingredient is most often sugar. The worst thing about fast food is that the more we eat it, the more we come to expect large amounts of sugar and salt in all of the foods we eat.

452. **Look for the increasingly popular fast-food outlets** that offer more healthful rotisserie-cooked chicken, turkey, and other home-style meals. Wholesome, low-sugar side dishes are also usually available at these eateries. Good choices to go with chicken and turkey include steamed, stewed, or baked vegetables, side salads, baked or mashed potatoes, roasted red potatoes, and sometimes even cooked sweet potatoes.

453. **Salad bars and a variety of prepackaged salads** are being offered at a number of outlets, including some of the bigger fast-food hamburger chains. If you know your schedule necessitates your picking up a salad to go, take along your own dressing (as described in bonus tip 438) to avoid the sugar-rich processed varieties.

454. **If for lunch you long for the food you eat at home,** invest in a wide-mouth Thermos and take food from home with you. Sugar-free soups and leftovers work particularly well in a Thermos, and they make for inexpensive lunches. It's also comforting to eat your favorite foods even when you're away from home.

455. **A Thermos also works well for making hot breakfast cereals** you can take with you in the morning or for making grain side dishes for trips and picnics. To make one serving of Thermos cereal, do what I do in a pinch: Pour in ⅓ cup of hot water and 2 tablespoons of buckwheat, millet, amaranth, or hot-water-soaked brown rice. Tighten the lid of the Thermos and let stand anywhere from half an hour to five hours. Add herbs, spices, milk, nuts, or fruit if desired, or eat as is from the container.

456. **Fat Flush Petite Pizzas,** explained in tip 272, are the ultimate sugar-free fast food.

457. **Whole food health bars,** such as StandardBars, are perfect light, chewy snacks and are free of sugar and artificial

sweeteners, providing a healthy alternative to the sugar-filled "health bars." The Berry StandardBar, for example, is a nutritious blend of three natural fruits—blueberries, cranberries, and cherries—that help to promote urinary tract health and are loaded with antioxidants. The bar provides an essential fatty acid (black currant seed oil) for immune support as well as added calcium for the central nervous system and the bones. The Peanut Butter StandardBar is a yummy, high protein, carb-controlled treat that will satisfy your cravings while providing your body with the powerful nutrition it needs for sustained energy. *Three sweet teeth.*
🦷 🦷 🦷

458. **When traveling by car,** pack some sugar-free snacks from home to avoid grabbing sugary snacks on the run. Peanut butter sandwiches, low-sugar granola bars, or nut-based trail mixes are three good choices. Review the tips in chapter 5 for other ideas.

459. **If you're traveling by plane, order a special meal** such as a diabetic, lacto-vegetarian, vegetarian, or cold seafood plate. A special meal does not guarantee that everything on your plate will be sugar-free, but it is usually a tremendous improvement over the standard meals. Place your order when you reserve your ticket, and be sure to double-check on your special meal a day before your departure.

460. **Also take high-quality snacks with you on the plane** because many flights don't serve meals anymore.

consumer alert
DON'T OVERLOOK THE SUGAR CONTENT
IN ENERGY BARS

In 2006 an estimated $600 million was spent on energy bars, according to SPINSscan data. In this fast-growing market, bars for energy, snacking, and weight management topped the list in sales. The kicker is that a random survey reported in the January/February 2007 Issue of *Nutraceuticals World* discovered that energy bar consumers were likely to over-look sugar content. While recent labeling requirement changes have helped to single out bars that are good sources of fats, consumers reported searching out protein, fiber, calcium, and antioxidants, yet seemed to overlook carbs, calories, and sugar. It is unclear whether this phenomenon is due to a fast-paced on-the-go lifestyle or labeling and marketing, but one thing is clear: you need to ask yourself, "Am I choos-ing a healthy snack or a dressed-up candy bar that over-shadows sugar content with vitamin and mineral labels?" In a market where taste rules and many stores have the narrow view of profit over product, you need to be sure of what is sweetening the product. Let's take a peek at some of the energy bars:

• **Oats 'n Honey Nature Valley Crunchy Granola Bars (General Mills)**
    Serving size: 1 packet (42 g) Calories 180
    Carbs 29 g Sugars 11 g

(continued)

- **Nutz over Chocolate Luna Bar (Clif Bar)**
  Serving size: 1 bar (48 g) Calories 180 Carbs 24 g
  Sugars 12 g

- **S'mores Luna Bar (Clif Bar)**
  Serving size: 1 bar (48 g) Calories 180 Carbs 27 g
  Sugars 12 g

- **Chocolate Chip Granola Optima Meal Bars (Slim-Fast Foods)**
  Serving size: 1 bar Calories 220 Carbs 35 g Sugars 15 g

- **Chocolate Cookie Dough Milk Chocolate Peanut Original Meal Bars/Meals-on-the-Go Bars (Slim-Fast Foods)**
  Serving size: 1 bar (56 g) Calories 220 Carbs 36 g
  Sugars 24 g

- **Trail Mix Chewy Granola Optima Meal Bars (Slim-Fast Foods)**
  Serving size: 1 bar Calories 210 Carbs 34 g Sugars 15 g

- **Vanilla Crisp Special K Bars (Kellogg)**
  Serving size: 1 bar (22 g) Calories 90 Carbs 17 g
  Sugars 7 g

- **Blueberry Nutri-Grain Cereal Bars (Kellogg)**
  Serving size: 1 bar (37 g) Calories 140 Carbs 26 g
  Sugars 13 g

- **Organic Fruits of Life Whole Food Antioxidant Matrix Bar (Garden of Life)**
  Serving size: 1 bar (64 g) Calories 230 Carbs 47 g
  Sugars 20 g

- **Atkins Advantage Wild Berry Granola Bar (Atkins)**
  Serving size: 1 bar (48 g) Calories 210 Carbs 18 g
  Sugars 1 g

Source: www.calorie-count.com

So what can you eat on the go? Remember, whole food health bars are free of sugar and artificial sweeteners (see tip 457). Some other bars worth noting are:

• **Power Bar's Pria Grain Essentials** are 70 percent organic with 8 grams per bar of whole grains, and they're made with inulin. Each bar contains 23 vitamins, 5–6 grams of protein, and a maximum of 3.5 grams of fat, with 40 percent of the daily value of calcium. They contain no artificial ingredients or coloring and no genetically modified ingredients.

• **Chocolate Almond Bliss**
   Serving size: 1 bar Calories 170 Carbs 29 g Sugars 8 g
   www.powerbarpria.com

• **T.H.E. Bar: Today's Health Equalizer** is a granola raisin bar that does not contain any high-fructose corn syrup, corn syrup, hydrogenated oils, or artificial sweeteners, flavors, or preservatives, plus it has no cholesterol. It is promoted as providing essential fatty acids and cardioprotective antioxidant nutrients as well as vitamins and minerals. Each bar contains 200 mg omega-3 fatty acids from ultra-refined fish oil, 900 mg pomegranate extract, 100 mg theaflavin-rich black tea extract, medium-chain triglycerides, and lecithin. It is also kosher dairy certified.

T.H.E. Bar (HVL, Inc.)
   Serving size: 1 bar (50 g) Calories 200 Carbs 25 g
   Sugars 10 g
   800-311-1950

High-protein snacks such as the Peanut Butter Standard-Bar (tip 457) are better for traveling than the honey-roasted nuts, muffins, or other sugary bites that airlines typically serve. I usually find snacks from home much more satisfying than airline food anyway. For the sugar-free hydration that is desperately needed when flying, I also like to take along bottled water.

get the sugar out of your mind and out of your life

*i*f you get the sugar out of your diet but continue to think about it every day and dream about it every night, the chances are not good that it will stay out of your diet for long.

That's because your beliefs, thoughts, and feelings really do have a huge impact on your actions. Current research into mind-body medicine shows that your thoughts even influence how your body physically perceives an experience. This means that if you work on altering your attitudes concerning sugar, your dietary transition away from sugar will be easier and more successful.

My experience with my clients seems to confirm the truth in these findings. I can tell you that the individuals who have made the most positive and lasting dietary changes were the ones who made life-changing attitudinal transformations as well.

Of course, changing misconceived ideas is only one part of

what is required to change long-standing eating habits. Other important parts are purely practical in nature—how you can get started, how you can stay motivated, and how you can cope with the physical, emotional, and social pressures that hold you back from changing.

This chapter covers these neglected but exceedingly important aspects to getting the sugar out. The tips include a potpourri of information, but these suggestions can sometimes make all the difference in helping you stick to an eating plan that keeps the sugar out.

Eating so as to keep the sugar out over the long term is the only way to maintain your best weight, and it is far better than going on and off nutritionally unsound fad diets. Tips to remind you of this—and tips that cover the importance of regular exercise—are also included in this chapter.

A decision to keep the sugar out of your life is a commitment to health that must last a lifetime. The tips that follow will help you keep this important commitment so your efforts will pay off in sweet rewards.

getting started

461. **Eliminate first the sugars that you are the least apt to miss:** those sugars that are hidden in drinks and in breakfast, lunch, and dinner convenience foods.

462. **Consult your doctor regularly** if you are currently taking medication. If you cut the sugar in your diet in a noticeable way, your cholesterol levels, blood pressure, or blood sugar

levels may change so dramatically that your medication may need to be reduced or perhaps eventually eliminated.

463. **Keep a food diary.** Jotting down everything you eat and drink for a few days is a surefire way of seeing the truth of your eating habits more clearly. Be sure to keep a record of what you eat on at least one weekend day, too, because you may eat irregularly and indulge in foods then that you don't usually have the rest of the week.

464. **Look for patterns in your food record**—in particular, when you crave and indulge in sweets. Several clients of mine who ate well the rest of the week were shocked at their sugar-craving mayhem on the weekends. Every weekend they went out for an unusually high-sugar breakfast: pancakes (made from white flour), high-sugar commercial pancake syrup, and a large glass of orange juice. This started a cycle that led to blood-sugar swings and sugar cravings and binges on those days.

465. **Make a bet to stay sugar-free.** You'd be amazed how sheer stubbornness and the desire to show the other person you can win the bet often give you unfailing resolve. (The opportunity to earn a little money doesn't hurt either.) A thirty-year-old career woman I know made a bet with her boss to give up chocolate for Lent. She had a difficult time not giving in to her desire for chocolate, but did it just to show him she could. The great thing was, after she won the bet, she felt so good, she decided not to go back to chocolate and to cut down on other forms of sugar as well!

466. Try staying sugar-free Vegas style. Find others who are trying to kick the sugar habit and encourage each person to bet money that both they and you can stick to a healthier, low-sugar lifestyle. If someone drops out, the rest of you get to split their money. Set the parameters so everyone clearly understands, and you'll be surprised by how well monetary bets keep you committed to getting the sugar out.

emotional considerations

467. Do not use sugar as a quick fix to help you cope with stress and tension. This is a common mistake. Eating sugar actually backfires: It depletes nutrient reserves, taxes the endocrine glands, and causes the body more stress, making you feel worse than you did before.

468. If you think sugar could not possibly have an effect on behavior, consider this: The brain controls our behavior, thought process, memory, learning, and moods. It is affected by any sudden changes in blood sugar because it uses almost half of all the available sugar in the blood. Studies have shown that excess sugar intake by children increases their likelihood of antisocial behavior, anxiety, lack of concentration, irritability, and emotional outbursts.

469. Be aware of the emotional factors behind when you desire sugar. See if you can make any connections between when you most want sugar and what types of things you are feeling then. If you find that you want sugar when you are most upset, talk to a trusted friend, meditate, take a relaxing bath, or try other ways to feel better that don't involve food.

470. **Don't fall into the trap of believing sugar will make you happy.** The pleasure you may experience from sugar on your taste buds is just temporary. It doesn't change any unhappiness you may be feeling from troubles with your friends, family, work, or love life. Remember, too, that sugar often causes depression and emotional upset, besides being a major contributor to the development of physical diseases that can affect us emotionally.

---

nutrient necessities

471. **Chromium, manganese, and zinc,** three trace minerals in short supply in the average American's diet, are needed to control blood sugar levels. Individuals with consistently low levels of these minerals are often diabetic. If you have hypoglycemia, diabetes, or any other type of blood sugar trouble, supplementation with these minerals is advisable. The usual daily dose is 200 to 600 of chromium, 10 to 30 of manganese, and 30 to 50 milligrams of zinc. Be sure the supplements you take are free of sugar.

472. **If you have intense cravings for sugar,** try taking 500 milligrams of the brain-feeding nutrient L-glutamine, up to three times per day. In the brain, L-glutamine converts to

glutamic acid, the only source of glucose besides sugar that the brain can use for energy. This amino acid is extremely helpful for people with hypoglycemia, and it has worked wonders for some of my most sugar-craving clients.

473. Support your adrenal glands for better blood sugar balance. The adrenals are constantly at work helping your body cope with such stresses as going too long without food or too much sugar. Since they are so important to blood sugar and health in general, be sure to nourish the adrenal glands with the vitamins and minerals they need—nutrients such as B-complex vitamins, pantothenic acid, vitamin C, zinc, and manganese. If you are stressed and your blood sugar is unbalanced, you might also want to consider taking adrenal and pancreatic glandular bovine tissue. With their RNA-DNA blueprints so similar to our own, these glandulars have proven extremely helpful for strengthening the adrenal and pancreatic function of many of my clients.

474. No matter how many nutrients you take, remember that sugar is an antinutrient that literally throws most of those nutrients down the toilet. Sugar is known to interfere with the absorption or increase the excretion of the B vitamins and almost all minerals. The best thing you can do to improve your nutrient status is not to take more supplements but to eat less sugar!

475. This is especially true for your calcium and magnesium levels. Both calcium and magnesium are excreted in the urine after sugar ingestion. No matter how much of these minerals you take in food and supplemental form, if you take them with a lot of sugar, you will not be able to absorb them. Since these minerals are crucial for strong bones, the huge rise in sugar intake may, in fact, be the primary reason for the high incidence of osteoporosis in the United States today.

the active ingredient

476. **If your discipline momentarily breaks down** and you eat some type of sweet concoction, don't despair. There's a simple solution: Exercise in whatever way you like best—walk, run, take a bike ride, play some tennis—so your body can use that sugar for energy instead of fat storage.

477. **Make social times active times.** Plan gatherings not around eating sugar but around exercise. For example, instead of meeting for coffee and dessert, schedule a tennis match or power walk or go out dancing.

478. **Why exercise regularly?** Because it's one of the most beneficial things you can do for your blood sugar and for your health. Regular exercise can lower blood sugar levels in diabetics and make insulin more effective for muscle and fat cells. It can also improve the body's absorption of nutrients, help prevent heart disease and osteoporosis, and increase the body's resistance to disease. In addition, regular exercise plays a key role in helping us look and feel our

best. It helps create a feeling of emotional well-being, relieving irritability, anxiety, and depression. Physically, it increases the body's endurance, muscle strength, and flexibility, and it promotes weight loss and weight control.

479. **You do not have to be a marathon runner to get the benefits of exercise.** Even a brisk twenty-minute walk four or more times a week will do. It does not matter so much at what level you start so long as you keep it up and gradually improve. Consistency is the key to receiving exercise's benefits.

480. **A little bit of a high-glycemic-index food** can give you a quick burst of energy for exercising, but don't use exercise as an excuse to overeat sugary foods. Too much sugar can even lessen the many beneficial effects of exercise.

slim for keeps

481. **Say no thanks to the latest unbalanced fad diet.** Starving yourself and living off grapefruit or sugar-rich "diet shakes" is not sensible, and the body knows it. A plan such as this may be a quick way to lose water weight and muscle mass, but it will do nothing for what you really want to lose—body fat. A fad starvation plan is also one of the quickest ways I know of to develop blood sugar problems and a slower body metabolism, both of which will almost certainly lead to more weight gain, not weight loss.

482. **Diet foods sweetened with aspartame are diet no-nos.** As already mentioned in tip 53, ingestion of aspartame (also known as NutraSweet or Equal) suppresses production of serotonin, a neurotransmitter that controls eating patterns. Without adequate serotonin, the body experiences intense sugar and carbohydrate cravings, which can lead to uncontrollable binge eating, which—guess what?— leads to more weight gain.

483. **Limit your carbohydrates to the level that is best for you.** Carbohydrate and sugar tolerance lessens with age and varies from individual to individual. For most people, a moderate intake of roughly 40 percent carbohydrates in their diets is more appropriate for health than a high-carbohydrate intake. Remember that too many carbohydrates in your system can lead to high levels of insulin, the fat-storage hormone. High insulin levels are probable precursors not only of obesity but also of heart disease, diabetes, and numerous other serious health conditions.

484. **An overlooked key to weight control** is maintaining a steady blood sugar level. Eating high-glycemic-index foods such as sugar may initially give you fast peaks in energy, but it will also cause a fast fall in blood sugar and energy that will leave you wanting more sugar later on. To maintain your blood sugar in the optimal zone for weight control, long-term energy, and health, emphasize instead low- and moderate-glycemic-index foods, foods that are as close to their natural state as possible, and a balance of high-quality protein, fat, and carbohydrates.

. . . .

485. **Get back to basics if you want to lose weight.** If you think about it, the most obvious and the safest way to promote weight loss is to avoid foods that give you unnecessary calories. Sugars, processed carbohydrates, and alcohol—which give you little of the nutrients you require—are the top three on that list.

486. **If you have tried every diet that there is** and have never experienced any permanent weight loss, understand that you need to give up the dieting game and adopt a sensible low-sugar eating plan for life. If you don't believe a lifelong low-sugar plan will benefit you in countless ways, I challenge you to try limiting the grains you consume to two servings per day and eating no more than 20 grams of sugar per day for one month. If you try this experiment, you might just be amazed at how your body responds.

---

the rest of the world

487. **Try going on a buddy system** with a friend who is also trying to cut the sugar out. The support and camaraderie from someone else with the same goals is often immeasurable.

488. **Or hire your own special buddy—a qualified nutritionist**—to help you with the practical ups and downs common with giving up sugar. A health professional trained

in nutrition can assist you with both the biochemical and emotional aspects of getting the sugar out as well as develop an individualized plan just for you.

489. **Be diplomatic but honest with your friends and relatives** and tell them that you would appreciate their not bringing sweets or spoiling your children with treats anymore. In a pleasant way, make it clear to them what you will allow and why you feel that way, and you might even get them to start thinking about going on their own sugar-lowering adventures!

490. **Also check with your children's day care providers and teachers** and make sure that sugar is not being used, as it often is, to pacify, reward, or discipline your children. Explain your feelings and most people will honor and respect them.

491. **Don't ever offer your child a sweet treat as a reward** to get him or her to eat. Doing so sets up an unhealthy situation and an even greater desire to indulge that sweet tooth.

492. **Prevent babies from developing an excessive sweet tooth** by not giving them nursing bottles full of fruit juice or water with honey or sugar in it. Giving children sweet drinks early in life sets the stage for tooth decay and promotes a strong desire for sweets that can lead to obesity later on.

493. **Enlist the assistance of your children** to help you find acceptable foods at the grocery store. Children are often willing to help, and if you make a game out of reading labels and finding good foods, they usually have fun responding to the challenge. They also learn a lot about food and how much sugar there is in food.

494. **Be creative when packing your school-age children's lunches.** Try to provide your children with healthful, fun, and nourishing treats that look so good their friends will want them too. The more you can accomplish this, the more your children will relish eating what you packed and not resort to the overly sweet, tooth-demolishing, mass-produced junk food available at so many schools today.

495. **All in the family? Why not?** Try to get others in your family to kick the sugar habit with you. It's much easier to stay away from sugar when the people close to you will also. Even if they won't, be sure they understand and respect just how important avoiding sugar is to you.

healthy attitudes, healthy life

496. **Don't get discouraged.** Persevere even when it seems as if all the people in the world (including your closest friends) are indulging their sweet tooth. You have to understand that you now know a secret many have yet to learn: Limiting your sugar intake is the key to better-looking skin, balanced moods, concentration, a trim physique, less

illness, and better all-around health. I myself find it much easier to go against the grain and keep the sugar out of my diet because I know that my efforts are paying off in how I look and feel today and will in the future.

497. **Concentrate on changing yourself for the better,** even when others close to you are not interested in doing the same. When others see how helpful getting the sugar out is for you, they might just follow your lead. Even if they don't, you need to remember that your primary responsibility in life is to be the best person that you can possibly be.

498. **Picture yourself being easily in control of the sugar you consume** and having a balanced, healthy attitude to food in general. Positive visualizations often translate into positive results.

499. **To ensure success, reinforce your commitment to eat for health** as much as you need. One person I know who had severe immune dysfunction posted this affirmation on her refrigerator to help her lick her sugar habit: "I want and deserve to take good care of myself. I can pass up sugar and be totally happy about it because I am replacing temporary, short-lived satisfaction in exchange for the greater satisfaction of long-term radiant health." (This meditation that she saw every day obviously worked. The woman is now free of her immunity problems.)

500. **Value yourself enough to nourish yourself with life-giving whole food.** Certain cultures, such as some Native

American tribes and the Chinese, believe that both plant-based and animal-based whole foods have a life force that strengthens our own life force when we eat them. When foods such as wheat and sugar are refined, however, the natural balance of minerals in these foods is destroyed, and they no longer supply the nutrition and the supportive energy they once did. Understanding this, you can choose unrefined foods over refined ones and take an important step toward better physical health and, consequently, better emotional, mental, and spiritual health as well.

501. **Treat yourself often to sweet experiences** in place of sweet food. Give yourself license to enjoy forgotten pleasures that don't revolve around food, such as soaking in a fragrant herbal bath, getting a relaxing massage, communing with nature, listening to uplifting music, buying yourself a long-awaited piece of clothing, or reading an adventure novel that takes you away for a while. When you allow yourself these kinds of healthy indulgences, sugar treats no longer seem necessary or desirable.

afterword

*e*arlier in my career, I went against traditional dietary wisdom when I wrote my first book, *Beyond Pritikin*, which became the foundation for the Fat Flush Plan. In that book, I explained how the right type of fat should not be avoided but rather included in the diet to promote optimal health. Now that health-conscious consumers such as you are starting to comprehend this message, it's high time you learn the equally important message that *sugar should be avoided* because it is, without a doubt, hazardous to human health. This book was written to remind you of this information and to show you practical ways to put this knowledge to work for you.

Facing up to the truth about sugar has not always been easy for me. I myself used to binge on sugar. I also know all too well how hard it is to avoid a substance that the rest of America holds in such high esteem.

But I had to start seeing the truth about sugar when my own father was diagnosed with adult-onset diabetes. Since there is a history of diabetes in my family and since diseases such as diabetes are linked to excessive sugar intake, I gradually began to realize that I had to get the sugar out of my diet to ensure my best health for the future.

More and more people are coming to this same conclusion. The evidence against sugar is simply too overwhelming to ignore.

Since you now know that eating too much sugar is tied to the most widespread and devastating illnesses of this century, act on what you know and limit your sugar consumption as the best way to maintain your health.

Sugar is finally being recognized as the villain it really is. As more research continues to uncover insulin and inflammation's roles in disease and aging, the dangers of excessive sugar in the diet will continue to be at the forefront of nutrition.

Our society will eventually catch up with current information about sugar, but until it does, be a trailblazer and use your sugar savvy for a healthy edge.

appendix

a week of sample menus

Here is a weeklong sample menu that incorporates the topics covered in *Get the Sugar Out*. The menu is designed to give you an idea of some of the things you can eat on a low-sugar eating plan for life.

As you can see, when you're on a health-maintenance diet such as this one, deprivation does not enter into the picture. You can have a wide variety of delicious food—even such treats as Danish pastries, cookies, and ice cream—as long as you choose your treats intelligently and incorporate them into a balanced diet.

This plan emphasizes the natural sugars in fresh vegetables and fruits and keeps intake of sugars to between 20 and 40 grams a day. Any level below 40 grams is a good goal for all of us to shoot for.

If, however, you are having trouble losing weight—or if you are recovering from diabetes, heart disease, cancer, parasites, yeast problems, or other health conditions—you should consider reducing sugars to below 20 grams per day. This level seems to allow maximum healing to take place and can be accomplished by substituting a serving of a low-starch vegetable (listed in tip 240) in place of any dessert or fruit listed on the menu.

This plan is just one example of how you can put the tips from this book into practice. The key to successful low-sugar eating is to use the sugar savvy you have developed to create a personal program that works for you.

MONDAY

Breakfast—1 Berry Nut Smoothie (tip 159)

Lunch—Salad plate with 1 cup romaine lettuce, ½ cup mixed baby greens, shredded red cabbage and carrot, and chopped tomato and cucumber, topped with 3 ounces of broiled seasoned chicken breast strips and 2 tablespoons vinegar-and-oil dressing

Dinner—Baked turkey meatballs made with 4 ounces ground turkey, oat bran, chopped onion, marjoram, and parsley; 1 serving Baked Spaghetti Squash (tip 222) with Fresh Pasta Sauce (tip 250)

TUESDAY

Breakfast—1 Peanut Butter StandardBar (tip 457)

Lunch—1 bean burrito made with ½ cup mashed pinto beans and one Fat Flush Tortilla, topped with chopped tomato, onion, shredded lettuce, ½ tablespoon guacamole with no sugar added, and 1 tablespoon salsa with no sugar added

Dinner—4 ounces broiled shrimp marinated in sesame oil, lime juice, garlic, and coriander; ½ cup spelt pasta topped with ½ cup zucchini, asparagus, and green onion sautéed in sesame or olive oil with fresh basil; 1 serving Vanilla Pears (tip 343) *or* ½ cup fresh pineapple tidbits topped with 1 tablespoon unsweetened shredded coconut

WEDNESDAY

Breakfast—1 hard-boiled egg; ½ cup Overnight Whole-Grain Cereal (tip 147) *or* 1 slice of sourdough rye toast

Lunch—1 peanut butter and apple sandwich with 2 tablespoons unsweetened peanut butter and thin slices of 1 fresh apple on 2 slices whole-grain bread

Dinner—1 serving Five-Spice Chicken and Vegetable Sauté (tip 234); ½ cup brown rice with 1 tablespoon Fat Flush West Indian Seasoning (tip 252); ¾ cup sliced fresh strawberries topped with a dollop of low-fat cultured yogurt mixed with a pinch of FOS-containing Flora-Key (tip 344) and a dash of natural vanilla extract (tip 345)

THURSDAY

Breakfast—1 Banana French Toast (tip 121) *or* 2 Sunburst Muffins (tip 118) spread with 1 tablespoon Peach Butter (tip 111), 1 tablespoon Carrot Butter (tip 112), *or* 1 teaspoon cinnamon-sprinkled butter (tip 105)

Lunch—Tuna salad made with 4 ounces of canned tuna, celery, green onion tops, water chestnuts, fresh lemon juice, and ½ tablespoon canola mayonnaise, served on Bibb lettuce or spinach leaves

Dinner—Roast Cornish game hen sprinkled with sage or thyme; ½ cup mixed green peas and carrots; ½ cup Brussels sprouts with 1 teaspoon butter

FRIDAY

Breakfast—1 orange; ½ cup oatmeal with 1 tablespoon raisins, 2 tablespoons chopped walnuts, and a sprinkling of ground cinnamon; served with 2 tablespoons whey protein powder plus 8 ounces water; 1 cup French Vanilla Café (tip 162)

Lunch—Hamburger made with ¼ pound broiled ground round served on a whole-grain spelt bun with lettuce, tomato, red onion slices, and 1 tablespoon Orange-Sesame Dressing (tip 185); 5 small jicama sticks

Dinner—4 ounces baked sole brushed with 1 teaspoon olive oil and fresh dill, served with a lemon wedge; 1 cup green beans almondine; 3 small Oatmeal Chocolate Chip Cookies (tip 396) *or* 1 serving Chocolate Ice Cream (tip 424)

SATURDAY

Breakfast—½ grapefruit; 2 poached eggs on 1 slice toasted HealthSeed spelt bread
Lunch—1 bowl Butternut Bisque (tip 173); 4 Sweetie Pie Flax Snack Crackers (tip 281)
Dinner—4 ounces roast turkey breast slices au jus; 1 small cooked sweet potato with 1 teaspoon butter; ½ cup steamed broccoli and cauliflower

SUNDAY

Brunch—5 Homemade Turkey Sausage patties (tip 140); 6 Melissa's Sweet Potato Pancakes (tip 129) topped with ¼ cup unsweetened peach applesauce
Snack—1 Fat Flush Petite Pizza (tip 272); 2 carrot strips and 2 celery sticks; 10 large fresh cherries
Dinner—4 ounces marinated and broiled lamb chop with ¼ cup Healthy Barbecue Sauce (tip 254); ⅓ cup long-grain brown rice, wild rice, and mushroom medley; side salad with red leaf lettuce, chopped tomato, cucumber, and 1 tablespoon French Olive Oil Dressing (tip 191)

Note: Remember to avoid sugars in the drinks you consume throughout the day. Choose any of the following sugar-free beverages both with meals and as mini-refreshers between meals: filtered water, mineral water, sparkling water, herbal teas, stevia-sweetened drinks, and FOS-sweetened drinks.

resources

ALLERGY RESOURCES
P.O. Box 888
Palmer Lake, CO 80133
719-488-3630
800-USE-FLAX

A mail order company that sells a wide selection of natural and alternative food and health products, including hard-to-find food items mentioned in this book such as maple syrup granules, date "sugar," fructose, FOS, and stevia. Call for a free catalog.

AMERICAN COLLEGE OF NUTRITION (ACN)
300 S. Duncan Avenue, Suite 225
Clearwater, FL 33755
727-446-6086
E-mail: office@amcollnutr.org
www.amcollnutr.org

The American College of Nutrition (ACN) was established in 1959 as a professional organization to promote scientific endeavor in the field of nutritional sciences. Its main goals are to enhance knowledge of nutrition and metabolism and the application of such knowledge to the maintenance of health and the treatment of disease. ACN provides an organization that encompasses the needs of professionals from all disciplines with a common interest in nutrition.

In addition, in 1993 ACN founded the Certification Board for Nutrition Specialists (CBNS) to help meet the growing demand for knowledgeable, responsible professional nutritionists. The

CBNS was created as a national certifying body in response to the many advanced-degree nutritionists (master's and doctoral level) from regionally accredited institutions that seek more formal recognition of their knowledge, skills, and experience. CBNS certification provides the public a way to distinguish highly trained, competent nutritionists with assurance. The CBNS Web site is www.cbns.org.

ASPARTAME CONSUMER SAFETY NETWORK

P.O. Box 2001
Frisco, TX 75034
214-387-4001
www.aspartamesafety.com

Aspartame Consumer Safety Network is an international non-profit organization consisting of thousands of volunteer health care professionals, scientists, and concerned consumers. The pioneer aspartame education and action organization was founded in 1987 by broadcast journalist and former state judge Mary Nash Stoddard and Washington, D.C., consumer advocate James Turner, Esq., in order to promote public awareness of a major health and public policy issue.

CLAYTON COLLEGE OF NATURAL HEALTH

2140 11th Avenue South, Suite 305
Birmingham, AL 35205
800-659-2426
205-323-8246
E-mail: communications@ccnh.edu
www.ccnh.edu

Clayton College of Natural Health (CCNH) offers college degree programs in natural health and holistic nutrition through distance education. These programs are designed to provide students with a wide variety of tools with which they can educate others in achieving and maintaining health through the use of natural elements, such as proper diet, pure water, clean air, exercise, and rest. In addition to degree programs in natural health and holistic nutrition, CCNH offers certificate and/or concentration programs in herbal studies, nutrition and lifestyles, and iridology.

FRENCH MEADOW BAKERY

2610 Lyndale Avenue South
Minneapolis, MN 55408
877-NO-YEAST
612-870-4740
www.frenchmeadowbakery.com

French Meadow Bakery offers the highest quality functional breads that are organic, dairy-free, yeast-free, and sugar-free. Perfect for the diabetic, vegetarian, vegan, and individuals who keep kosher. Look for French Meadow breads (including the HealthSeed Spelt and Fat Flush Tortilla) in the refrigerated and frozen natural bread section in your local health food store or in specialty supermarkets.

THE NATIONAL ASSOCIATION OF NUTRITION PROFESSIONALS (NANP)

P.O. Box 1172
Danville, CA 94526

Phone 800-342-8037
Fax 510-580-9429
www.nanp.org

The National Association of Nutrition Professionals (NANP) is a nonprofit business league of nutrition professionals originally founded in 1985 as the Society of Certified Nutritionists. The NANP represents holistically trained nutrition professionals. Their mission is to enhance the integrity of the holistic nutrition profession through self-governance, educational standards, a rigorous code of ethics, and professional registration of holistic nutritionists.

FIRST FOR WOMEN
270 Sylvan Avenue
Englewood Cliffs, NJ 07632
800-938-8312
www.firstforwomen.com

This magazine speaks directly to women about their real-life needs, concerns, and interests. I have been the nutrition columnist for *First for Women* since 2003. Do check out my monthly "Nutrition Know-How."

HEALTH SCIENCES INSTITUTE
702 Cathedral Street
Baltimore, MD 21201
888-213-0764
E-mail: hsiresearch@healthiernews.com
www.hsibaltimore.com

As a member of the professional advisory panel, I can verify that this cutting-edge newsletter is devoted to presenting extraordinary products to its members before the products hit the marketplace. The Health Sciences Institute provides private access to hidden cures, powerful discoveries, breakthrough treatments, and advances in modern, underground medicine.

TASTE FOR LIFE

86 Elm Street
Petersborough, NH 03458
603-924-9692
E-mail: customerservice@tasteforlife.com
www.tasteforlife.com

This is one of the fastest growing in-store magazines for health food stores, natural product chains, food co-ops, and supermarkets nationwide. Its excellent articles on pertinent health issues offer readers an informative educational source on a variety of levels, including physical fitness. I sit on *Taste for Life*'s editorial board.

TOTAL HEALTH MAGAZINE FOR LONGEVITY

165 North 100 East, Suite 2
St. George, Utah 84770-2205
888-316-6051
435-673-1789
E-mail: thm@infowest.com
www.totalhealthmagazine.com

I am fortunate to serve as an associate editor for this magazine. It is a comprehensive voice in antiaging, longevity, and self-managed natural health. Lyle Hurd, publisher extraordinaire, strives to bring readers fresh new information and perspectives on all phases of longevity medicine so that you can make an educated decision on the quality of your life today . . . and tomorrow.

UNI KEY HEALTH SYSTEMS, INC.
181 West Commerce Drive
P.O. Box 2287
Hayden Lake, ID 83835
Sales: 800-888-4353
Service: 208-762-6833
Fax: 208-762-9395
E-mail: unikey@unikeyhealth.com
www.unikeyhealth.com

To make shopping easier and more convenient, Uni Key Health Systems has distributed supplements to my clients and readers for over fifteen years. For example, Uni Key carries Flora-Key, mentioned in this book (Tip 71), as well as many of the books from which my recipes are derived. By calling Uni Key directly, you can special order StandardBars.

WIKIPEDIA
www.wikipedia.com

Since its creation in 2001, Wikipedia has rapidly grown into the largest reference Web site on the Internet. The content of Wikipedia is free and is written collaboratively by people from all around the world. This Web site is a wiki, which means that *anyone* with access to an Internet-connected computer can edit, correct, or improve information throughout the encyclopedia, simply by clicking the "Edit This Page" link (with a few minor exceptions, such as protected articles and the main page).

Wikipedia is a registered trademark of the nonprofit Wikimedia Foundation, which has created an entire family of wiki projects. On Wikipedia and its sister projects, you are welcome to be bold and edit articles yourself, contributing knowledge as you see fit in a collaborative way.

bibliography

Abrahamson, E. M., and A. W. Pezet. *Body, Mind and Sugar.* New York: Holt, Rinehart and Winston, 1951.

Allman, William F. "Aspartame: Some Bitter with the Sweet?" *Science* 84, 5 (July/August 1984): 14.

Appleton, Nancy. *Lick the Sugar Habit.* Garden City Park, N.Y.: Avery Publishing Group, 1988.

Atkins, Robert C. *Dr. Atkins' New Diet Revolution.* New York: M. Evans and Company, 1992.

Barkie, Karen E. *Sweet and Sugarfree.* New York: St. Martin's Press, 1982.

Blaylock, Russell. *Excitotoxins: The Taste That Kills.* Santa Fe, N.M.: Health Press, 1994.

Blumenthal, Mark. "Is Stevia Too Sweet for Us?" *Let's Live,* June 1992, 66–67.

Buhr, Deborah E. *The "I Can't Believe This Has No Sugar" Cookbook.* New York: St. Martin's Press, 1990.

Burrows, Nancy. *Allergy Cooking Tricks and Treasures.* Grand Forks, N.D.: Nancy Burrows, 1987.

Challem, Jack, Burt Berkson, and Melissa Diane Smith. *Syndrome X.* New York: John Wiley and Sons, Inc.

Cleave, T. L. *The Saccharine Disease.* New Canaan, Conn.: Keats Publishing, 1975. "The Confectionery Elite 1994." *Confectioner,* May/June 1995.

Crayhon, Robert. *Health Benefits of FOS (Fructooligosaccharides).* New Canaan, Conn.: Keats Publishing, 1995.

———. *Robert Crayhon's Nutrition Made Simple.* New York: M. Evans and Company, 1994.

Crook, William G. *The Yeast Connection and the Woman*. Jackson, Tenn.: Professional Books, 1995.

Crook, William G., and Marjorie Hurt Jones. *The Yeast Connection Cookbook*. Jackson, Tenn.: Professional Books, 1989.

Dufty, William. *Sugar Blues*. New York: Warner Books, 1975.

Fredericks, Carlton, and Herman Goodman. *Low Blood Sugar and You*. New York: Grosset and Dunlap, 1969.

Gittleman, Ann Louise. *Beyond Pritikin*. New York: Bantam Books, 1996.

———. *Hot Times*. New York: Avery, 2005.

———. *The Fast Track Detox Diet*. New York: Morgan Road Books, 2006.

———. *The Fat Flush Cookbook*. New York: McGraw-Hill, 2003.

———. *The Fat Flush Plan*. New York: McGraw-Hill, 2001.

———. *Super Nutrition for Women*. Revised and updated edition. New York: Bantam Books, 2004.

———. *Eat Fat, Lose Weight Cookbook*. New York: McGraw-Hill, 2001.

———. *Your Body Knows Best*. New York: Pocket Books, 1996.

Goldbeck, Nikki and David. *The Good Breakfast Book*. Woodstock, N.Y.: Ceres Press, 1992.

Horner, Christine. *Waking the Warrior Goddess*. New Jersey: Basic Health Publishing, 2005.

Hull, Janet Starr. *Sweet Poison*. Far Hills, N.J.: New Horizon Press, 1998.

———. *Splenda: Is It Safe or Not*. McKinney, Tex.: Pickle Press, 2005.

Hunt, Douglas. *No More Cravings*. New York: Warner Books, 1987.

Hyman, Mark. *Ultra Metabolism*. New York: Scribner, 2006

Jones, Jeanne. *Cook It Light*. New York: Macmillan, 1987.

Kamen, Betty. *The Chromium Diet, Supplement and Exercise Strategy.* Novato, Calif.: Nutrition Encounter, Inc., 1990.

Kinderlehrer, Jane. *Smart Breakfasts.* New York: Newmarket Press, 1989.

Krohn, Jacqueline, et al. *The Whole Way to Allergy Relief and Prevention.* Point Roberts, Wash.: Hartley and Marks, 1991.

Kuczmarski, Robert J., et al. "Increasing Prevalence of Overweight Among U.S. Adults." *Journal of the American Medical Association* 272 (1994): 205–11.

Mason, Michael. "Confessions of a Fat-Free Snack Junkie." *Health,* May/June 1995, 36, 42.

Melos, Linda. *Sugar and Carbohydrate Intolerance.* Phoenix, Ariz.: Eck Institute, 1987.

Mindell, Earl. *Safe Eating.* New York: Warner Books, 1987.

Nostrand, Carol A. *Junk Food to Real Food.* New Canaan, Conn.: Keats Publishing, 1994.

O'Neill, Molly. "So It May Be True After All: Eating Pasta Makes You Fat." *New York Times,* February 8, 1995.

Quillin, Patrick. *Beating Cancer with Nutrition.* Tulsa, Okla.: Nutrition Times Press, 1994.

Phelps, Janice Keller, and Allan E. Nourse. *The Hidden Addiction and How to Get Free.* Boston: Little, Brown, 1986.

Schauss, Alexander. *Diet, Crime and Delinquency.* Berkeley, Calif.: Parker House, 1981.

Spiller, Gene. *The Superpyramid Eating Program.* New York: Random House, 1993.

Townsley, Cheryl. *Kids' Favorites.* Littleton, Colo.: Cheryl Townsley, 1992.

Yudkin, John. *Sweet and Dangerous.* New York: Wyden Books, 1972.

permissions

"Almond Milk" from *Hot Times: How to Eat Well, Live Healthy, and Feel Sexy During the Change* by Ann Louise Gittleman. Copyright © 2005 by Ann Louise Gittleman. Reprinted by permission of Avery, a division of Penguin Group Inc.

"Almond-Oat Squares" adapted from "Sesame-Oat Squares" from *The Yeast Connection Cookbook* by William G. Crook, M.D., and Marjorie Hurt Jones. Copyright © 1989 by William G. Crook, M.D., and Marjorie Hurt Jones. Reprinted by permission of Professional Books.

"Apple, Cranberry, and Pear Crisp" from *Hot Times: How to Eat Well, Live Healthy, and Feel Sexy During the Change,* by Ann Louise Gittleman. Copyright © 2005 by Ann Louise Gittleman. Reprinted by permission of Avery, a division of Penguin Group Inc.

"Avocado-Cilantro Dip" from *Eat Fat Lose Weight Cookbook,* by Ann Louise Gittleman. Copyright © 2001 by Ann Louise Gittleman. Reprinted by permission of McGraw-Hill.

"Baked Sweet Beans" from *Healing with Whole Foods: Oriental Traditions and Modern Nutrition,* by Paul Pitchford. Copyright © 1993, 1996 by Paul Pitchford. Reprinted by permission of Atlantic Books, Berkeley, California.

"Banana Cheesecake in a Cup" from *Hot Times: How to Eat Well, Live Healthy, and Feel Sexy During the Change,* by Ann Louise Gittleman. Copyright © 2005 by Ann Louise Gittleman. Reprinted by permission of Avery, a division of Penguin Group Inc.

"Catherine's Favorite Chocolate Cake." Reprinted by permission of Chatfield's Company.

"Chewy Banana-Oat Cookies" from *Allergy Cooking Tricks and Treasures* by Nancy Burrows. Copyright © 1987 by Nancy Burrows. Reprinted by permission of Nancy Burrows. For more information write to: *Allergy Cooking Tricks and Treasures,* 8050 Downing Drive, Denver, CO 80229.

"Chocolate-Coated-Fruit Party Platter" from *The All-Natural Sugar Free Dessert Cookbook* by Linda Romanelli Leahy. Copyright © 1992 by Lynn Sonberg Book Services. Reprinted by permission of Dell Books, a division of Bantam Doubleday Dell Publishing Group, Inc.

"Chocolate Ice Cream" from *The "I Can't Believe This Has No Sugar" Cookbook* by Deborah Buhr. Copyright © 1990 by Deborah Buhr. Reprinted by permission of St. Martin's Press, Inc., New York, New York.

"Crispy Unfried Chicken" from *The Fat Flush Cookbook,* by Ann Louise Gittleman. Copyright © 2003 by Ann Louise Gittleman. Reprinted by permission of McGraw-Hill.

"Crispy Unfried Fish" from *The Fat Flush Cookbook,* by Ann Louise Gittleman. Copyright © 2003 by Ann Louise Gittleman. Reprinted by permission of McGraw-Hill.

"Everything Good Birthday Cake" adapted from *Eating for A's,* by Alexander Sehauss, Barbara Friedland Meyer, and Arnold Meyer. Reprinted by permission of Pocket Books.

"Fabulous Flaxy Crackers" from *The Fast Track Detox Diet,* by Ann Louise Gittleman. Copyright © 2005 by Ann Louise Gittleman. Reprinted by permission of Morgan Road Books.

"Famous Spaghetti Squash Pudding with Mixed Berry Puree." Reprinted by permission of Barbara Anderson, one of my ardent Fat Flushers.

"Fat Flush Lemonade" from *The Fat Flush Cookbook,* by Ann Louise Gittleman. Copyright © 2003 by Ann Louise Gittleman. Reprinted by permission of McGraw-Hill.

"Fat Flush Petite Pizza" from *The Fat Flush Cookbook,* by Ann Louise Gittleman. Copyright © 2003 by Ann Louise Gittleman. Reprinted by permission of McGraw-Hill.

"Fat Flush West Indian Seasoning" from *The Fat Flush Cookbook,* by Ann Louise Gittleman. Copyright © 2003 by Ann Louise Gittleman. Reprinted by permission of McGraw-Hill.

"Five-Spice Chicken and Vegetable Sauté" from *Beyond Pritikin* by Ann Louise Gittleman. Copyright © 1988 by Ann Louise Gittleman. Reprinted by permission of Bantam Books, a division of Bantam Doubleday Dell Publishing Group, Inc.

"French Olive Oil Dressing" from *Beyond Pritikin,* by Ann Louise Gittleman. Copyright © 1988 by Ann Louise Gittleman. Reprinted by permission of Bantam Books, a division of Bantam Doubleday Dell Publishing Group, Inc.

"Fresh Pasta Sauce." Reprinted by permission of Holly J. Sollars.

index

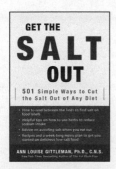
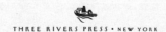

- Whole-grain crackers
- Cheese
- ~~Cinna~~ Cinnamon stick